IMPORTANT FACTS
ABOUT CANCER PREVENTION

Dr. Abdelfattah Mohsen Badawi

Order this book online at www.trafford.com
or email orders@trafford.com

Most Trafford titles are also available at major online book retailers.

Printed in the United States of America.

ISBN: 978-1-4669-5359-8 (sc)
ISBN: 978-1-4669-5361-1 (hc)
ISBN: 978-1-4669-5360-4 (e)

Library of Congress Control Number: 2012915041

Trafford rev. 08/16/2012

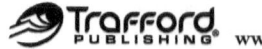 www.trafford.com

North America & international
toll-free: 1 888 232 4444 (USA & Canada)
phone: 250 383 6864 ♦ fax: 812 355 4082

Contents

Acknowledgement

This book IMPORTANT FACTS ABOUT CANCER PREVENTION was commissioned by Professor Abdelfattah M Badawi.

The editing of the chapters as submitted and the arranging of the text and chapters in all cases was carried out under the guidance of Professor Nadia G Kandile. Considerable thanks must be expressed to Professor Kandile for their efforts in producing this book in a form ready for publication. Professor David RK Harding's assistance is also acknowledged.

A Tribute To My Late Wife, M.Sc Chemist, Shahira Alshishini

She was born Shahira on April 29th, 1946 in Alexandria. She graduated from Lycee France High School in 1962. I first have seen her on summer 1962 when she was 16 years old at Abuhave sea shore and when I asked to marry her, her family refused as she was so young. She was the most beautiful girl I had ever seen.

After five years seeing so many girls and by mere accident, when on year 1967 I was going to Faculty of Science, Ain Shams University, I have seen her going out from a course for MSc Chemistry and she was 21 years old. I tried talk to her but she was disappointed as she was just has been separated from her fiancé in USA and refused to go to him. For 2 months, I insisted to contact her and at last approved that I go to her father Professor Alshishini at the National Academy of Science in Cairo. I met him several times and at last he approved to engage his daughter. She became my fiancé or one year and during that time she told me that she feels that she will die young.

I always thought she was the most beautiful woman I had ever seen. This is how I always saw her and will always remember her. Here is our wedding picture taken on the 11th April, 1968 when she was 22 years old.

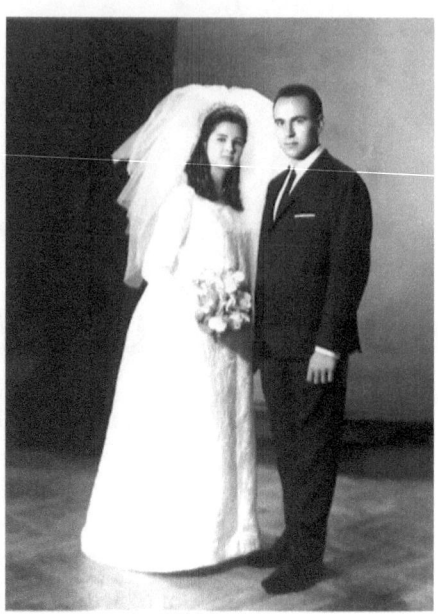

Shahira was a vibrant, determined, and creative person. She had her own thoughts and was not afraid to express them. Over the years she worked as a chemist at the Institute of Chemistry for Quality Control Testing at the Ministry of Industry, Cairo, Egypt.

During all this time Shahira had better physical fitness than me especially during swimming in Alexandria at Mediterranean Sea. But she was very worried when she got her period each month indicating no pregnancy. Medical inspection showed no obstacles for her pregnancy at all.

After five years (1973) she got permanent cough and pain inside her chest. Checking her case with well known consulting doctors in Cairo, they advised us to go the Gustave Russi Hospital in Paris. Her father, mother and I traveled to France

In hospital her case was diagnosed as non-Hodgkin disease exerting lymphoma inside her chest. She got radiotherapy for 4 months and we were recommended to check up, here she is at the age of 27. We had been married for six years at the time.

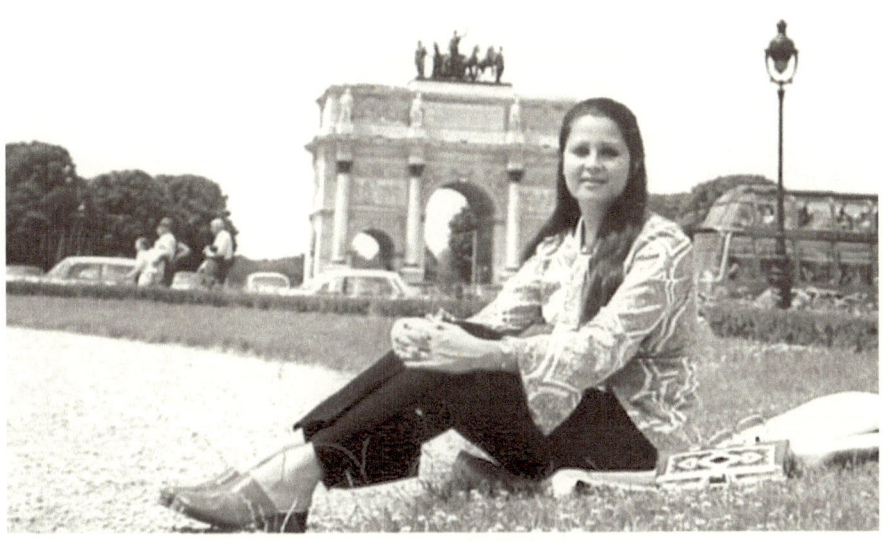

She returned home in Cairo and after one year. The cough began to attack her. Returning back to France, her doctor recommended chemotherapy and she began treatment after returning back to Cairo.

She insisted to enjoy our summer holiday in August 1974 at Marsa Matroh beach, West of Alexandria. After returning from this holiday, her cough returned. In December 1974, her case deteriorated and she was hospitalized and passed away on 27th January, 1975.

This book I dedicate to the memory of my beloved Shahira.

Abdelfattah Badawi

Preface

Cancer is a global epidemic. In 2008, it was estimated there were 12,332,300 cancer cases of which 5.4 million were in developed countries and 6.7 million were in developing countries. Over half of the incident cases occurred in residents of four WHO regions. The world population increased from 6.1 billion in 2000 to 6.7 billion in 2008. The increase in populations was much more in developing countries than in developed countries. Even if the age-specific rates of cancer remain constant, developing countries would have a higher cancer burden than developed countries.

Cancer trends are showing upward trends in many developing countries and a mixed pattern in developed countries. By 2050, the cancer burden could reach 24 million cases per year worldwide, with 17 million cases occurring in developing countries. Cancers which are associated with diet and life style are seen more in developed countries while cancers which are due to infections are more in developing countries. According to the World Health Organization (WHO), death from cancer is expected to increase to 104% worldwide by 2020. While the number of total cancer cases is increasing, the trend of certain cancers is changing in developed and developing countries.

Cancer is a multi-step process typically occurring over an extended period beginning with initiation followed by promotion and progression. Often cancers arise due to over expression of oncogenes or expression of inappropriate protein products produced by gene translocations, insertions, or rearrangements.

Cancer is a complex disease occurring as a result of a progressive accumulation of genetic and epigenetic changes that enable escape from normal cellular and environmental control. Cancer is a generic term for a group of more than 100 diseases that can affect any part of the body. Other terms used are malignant tumors and neoplasms. One defining feature of cancer is the rapid creation of abnormal cells which grow beyond their usual boundaries and which can invade adjoining parts of the body and spread to other organs, a process referred to as metastasis. Metastases are the major cause of death from cancer.

Cancer is the result of a multistep process in which the cumulative effect of successive genetic and molecular alterations leads to a gradual transition, typically over decades, from normal to increasing grades of dysplasia that culminate in an invasive and metastatic phenotype.

The sequential accumulation of genetic and molecular alterations over time provides opportunities for the development of clinical interventions aimed at both preventing cancer initiation and at treating premalignant lesions.

Cancer is a disease, or some believe a set of diseases, characterized by a population of cells that grow and divide without respect to normal limits, invade and destroy adjacent tissues and may spread to distant anatomic sites. Nearly all cancers are caused by abnormalities in the genetic material of the transformed cells. These abnormalities may be due to the effects of the environment, such as exposure to carcinogens, or cancer-promoting genetic abnormalities which may be inherited and thus present in all cells from birth.

Complex interactions between carcinogens and the host genome make it a challenging task for researchers to understand the underlying mechanism of action and find cures for the many forms of this disease. Thus, it is important for researchers to have tools that allow them to easily study cancerous cells and their affects under varying biological conditions.

For instance, researchers want to understand how cancerous cells bypass the natural process of programmed cell death or apoptosis, as well as how some genes may exert control over the cell cycle to encourage or prevent unwanted cell growth.

Cancer continues to represent the largest cause of mortality in the world and claims over 6 million lives each year. An extremely promising strategy for cancer prevention today is chemoprevention, which is defined as the use of synthetic or natural agents (alone or in combination) to block the development of cancer in human beings. Plants, vegetables, herbs and spices used in folk and traditional medicine have been accepted currently as one of the main sources of cancer chemopreventive drug discovery and development.

Today, cancer is recognized as a highly heterogeneous disease and over 100 distinct types have been described with various tumor subtypes found within specific organs. It is now also recognized that genetic and phenotypical variability primarily determines the self-progressive growth, invasiveness and metastatic potential of neoplastic disease and its response or resistance to therapy. It seems that this multi-level complexity of cancer explains the clinical diversity of histologically similar neoplasias.

Recent advances in other disciplines have uncovered that in addition to virus infection, disregulation of many normal cellular processes such as gene regulation, cell cycle control, DNA repair and replication, checkpoint signaling, differentiation and apoptosis can lead to cancer. The mechanisms of transformation can be complex with multiple pathways affected. For example, genetic changes in the p53 gene resulting in loss of heterozygosity are known to affect the pattern of gene activation and repression, dampen cell cycle checkpoints and incapacitate the induction of apoptosis.

Cancer chemoprevention is a mean of cancer control by pharmacological intervention of the occurrence of the disease using chemical compounds.

Recent events suggest that new emphasis in the development of medical treatment of human disease will be intimately connected to natural products. The use of medicinal plants in modern medicine for the prevention or treatment of cancer is an important aspect. For this reason, it is important to identify anti-tumor promoting agents present in medicinal plants commonly used by the human population which can inhibit the progression of tumors.

Chemoprevention can be defined as the use of natural or chemically synthesized compounds to prevent, inhibit or reverse the process of carcinogenesis. The concept of chemoprevention gained momentum when numerous laboratory studies showed anticancer effects of natural agents in various tumor models. However, natural agents failed to prove their worth at the last and most expensive step, i.e. in the clinic. Many reasons have been attributed to this failure that range from lack of clearly defined mechanism of action to poor bioavailability. Further, the observed anti-cancer activity of different natural agents in cell culture and animal models does not translate into clinically beneficial outcome in humans. This is because laboratory studies tend to investigate pharmacological effects at doses that are not achievable in humans through dietary sources. Based on these important and limiting factors, the science of chemoprevention has less proponents and more critics. Nevertheless since, the term chemoprevention was coined 40 years ago, researchers through extensive high throughput screening have identified an arsenal of anticancer drugs from natural sources.

Chemoprevention is an innovative area of cancer research that focuses on the prevention of cancer through pharmacologic, biologic and nutritional intervention. As originally described, this involves the primary prevention of initiation and the secondary prevention, delay or reversal of promotion and progression. Several agents have demonstrated cancer preventive risk reduction in large phase 3 clinical trials in individuals with an increased risk of cancer. Other large trials are ongoing.

There are several possible approaches to cancer prevention. Patients can decrease behaviors that put them at risk, be more vigilant in screening and surveillance, opt for surgical pre-intervention and/or utilize "medicinal" approaches. The latter three areas in particular can benefit from the advances that nanotechnology can offer.

It is well recognized that several factors contribute to and enhance cancer prevention including dietary and lifestyle changes. The field of epidemiology has long been examining what types of risk factors are correlated with certain types of cancers. For instance, probably one of the best documented and most studied behavioral risk factors is that smoking increases the incidence of lung cancer. In fact, smoking also greatly increases the risk of many types of cancers as well as heart attacks. A second well documented example is increased exposure to UVB rays from sunlight clearly damages DNA and can result in an increased risk of various types of skin cancer including the most deadly, melanoma.

This book was conceived with the idea of focusing on one a many worldwide research programs and that is the role of different agents in the war against cancer. Metals and metal compounds have been used in medicine for several thousands of years. In this book, we present a selection of anti-cancer activities and cancer prevention potential for a selection of metal ions.

This book comprises 10 chapters dealing with variegated aspects of cancer and prevention. The chapters covered the role of many topics in cancer prevention as chemical carcinogenesis, some natural and synthetic compounds, metal ions, metals, trace elements, amino acids, surfactants and nanotechnology.

Now comes the pleasant task of thanking those who contributed towards materialization of this book. We are especially thankful to all the contributors for their interest, enthusiasm and cooperation without which this book would not have seen the light of day.

Dr Nadia G. Kandile
Professor of Applied Chemistry, Department of Chemistry
Faculty of Women, Ain Shams University
Heliopolis, 1175
Cairo, Egypt

The Ascorbic Acid Molecule in OrthomolecularTherapy and Prevention of Cancer.
A Recent Review

Dr Abdelfattah Badawi

General Secretary for the International Society of Therapeutic,
Experimental and Clinical Research (Bastia, France).
Professor, Applied Surfactant Laboratory,
Egyptian Petroleum Research Institute, Nasr City, Cairo, Egypt.

Introduction

Ascorbic acid (AA) plays an important role in oxidative stress control. AA in combination with other nutrients promotes normal metabolism and they interact with each other to facilitate absorption within the body. Most cancer patients die with nutritional imbalances that are difficult to correct by dietary intake alone. An AA questionnaire together with specific laboratory panels of biological tests can be implemented for cancer patients. These tools may serve to provide data for assessing the patient's AA oxidative stress, clinical status and directing AA intervention to alleviate treatment related complications. This may result in improved quality of life, decreased morbidity and prolonged survival. This review will provide an update of peer reviewed scientific data related to the impact and outcome of orthomolecular AA on cancer therapy and prevention.

Orthomolecular oncology

There are a wide variety of mechanisms by which AA prevents and inhibits malignant growth. The collective evidence supports the notion of increasing AA intake in patients suffering malignancies, especially if provided by the intra venous route. AA may produce benefits in both prevention and treatment of cancer by inhibiting malignant cell proliferation and inducing differentiation. [1] The ideal anticancer agent is obviously one that specifically interferes with tumor growth, prolongs patient survival time and improves the patient's quality of life. There is evidence that AA might fit this description. Based on this evidence, it is suggested that the use of intra venous AA as an advent therapy in cancer treatment be promoted. [2]

Orthomolecular AA as therapy for human cancer

Mehdavi et al., [3] have determined the levels of oxidative stress, serum total antioxidants and AA in a cohort of 57 cancer patients and 22 healthy participants. The level of oxidative stress was measured by malondialdehyde (the end product of lipid peroxidation). Cancer patients as compared with controls, showed a significant increase in lipid peroxidation with a concomitant decrease in the antioxidant defense system. In addition, low serum levels of AA in spite of adequate daily intake may be because of increased use of scavenging lipid peroxides as well as their sequestration by tumor cells.

The effect of chemotherapy alone versus a high dose of AA (6100mg/d) combined with vitamin E (1050mg/d) and β-carotene (60 mg/d) in patients with advanced non small cell lung cancer (NSCLC) indicated a potential benefit for AA. [4] Frei and Lawson reported the potential of AA as therapy for human cancer. [5] The authors are located at the Linus Pauling Institute and they revitalized interest in AA promoted by the investigations of Cameron and Pauling (Noble laureate) that led to their conclusion "*that treatment with AA in amounts of 10g/day or more is of real value in extending the life of patients with advanced cancer*". [6]

Frei and Lawson stressed the high statistical significance of the positive effect of AA and stated that "*a series of case reports indicated that high-dose AA was associated with long-term tumor regression in three patients with advanced renal cell carcinoma, bladder carcinoma, or B-cell lymphoma*". [7]

AA with nutrient mixture inhibits human bladder and adenocarcinoma cell lines

A nutrient mixture (NM) of AA, lysine, proline, arginine and green tea extract was reported to inhibit human bladder cancer cells and the human T-24 adenocarcinoma line 760-0. [8,9] The invasion of both human cancer cells was totally inhibited by a NM at 1000 microgram/ml. Highly metastatic melanoma is resistant to existing therapies. Mice supplemented with NM not only showed less tumor growth in the spleen in control mice but also drastically reduced metastasis to the liver. [10] Strengthening of collagen and connective tissue can be achieved naturally through the synergistic effects of NM. The NM used exhibited a potent anticancer activity in vivo and in vitro in low dose cancer cell lines. The NM anticancer effects include inhibition of metastasis tumor growth, matrix metalloproteinase (MMP) secretion, invasion, angiogenesis and cell growth as well as induction of apoptosis. [11]

AA administered intra venously as a cancer therapy

The history of AA and cancer has been marked with controversy. Clinical studies evaluating AA as a viable anticancer therapeutic continue to the present day. However, the wealth of data suggesting that AA may be highly beneficial in addressing cancer associated inflammation, particularly progression to systemic inflammatory response syndrome (SIRO) and multi organ failure (MOF) have been largely overlooked. Patients with advanced cancer are generally deficient in AA. Once these patients develop septic symptoms, a further decrease in ascorbic acid levels occurs. Given the known role of ascorbate in a) maintaining endothelial and suppression of inflammatory markers, b) protection from sepsis in animal models and c) direct antineoplastic effects, we propose the use of AA as an adjuvant to existing modalities in the treatment and prevention of cancer associated sepsis. [12]

AA and vitamin K3 as cancer therapy

A combination of AA and quinine was used as a supplemental treatment for an ovarian cancer patient. The combination may be administered before, during and after the patient undergoes a conventional cancer treatment protocol. The combination may be administered orally, intravenously, or intraperitoneally. Oral administration may be in the form of capsules containing a predetermined ratio of AA to Vitamin K_3. The supplemental treatment is effective to inhibit metastases of cancer cells and inhibit tumor growth. The ratio the AA to Vitamin K_3 is in the range of about 50 to 1 to about 250 to 1. A method for evaluating the effectiveness of the supplemental treatment includes monitoring the patient's serum DNase activity throughout the course of treatment. [13]

AA and metal ions as catalytic cancer therapy

In catalytic therapy (CT), most often the combination of AA as a substrate and phthalocyanine dyes containing transition metal ions as catalysts is used. Mechanisms underlying the antitumor action of CT are similar to X-ray therapy and photodynamic therapy (PDT) cancer treatments, in that CT actions are dependent on the production of reactive oxygen species (ROS). ROS subsequently induce oxidative degradation of critical cellular molecules and organelles. [14-17] Compared to traditional chemotherapy and PDT, CT has the potential to become a preferred treatment for an array of diverse malignancies. It has been found that a combination of cobalt or iron phthalocanine and sodium ascorbate has high antitumor activity. This system is highly effective with a success rate similar to that of PDT. The effectiveness of CT has been demonstrated in *in vitro* experiments with porphyrin-like moieties (vitamin B12) and its derivatives as catalysts with ascorbate as a substrate.

[18-20] Several in vivo experiments with the same CT systems have also been reported. [21-24] A combination of teraphthal (cobalt (II) octa-4, 5-carboxyphthalocyanine) and AA was approved for Phase II clinical trials in Russia. [25] AA is currently considered the most suitable substrate for CT. It has been well recognized that some human tumors accumulate AA more readily than normal tissues do. It has also been demonstrated that AA may be a prodrug for the formation of H_2O_2 in tumor cells. [26] In addition, formation of H_2O_2 and $OH^-$by photosensitizers such as methylene blue, hematoporphyrin, and texaphyrines in the presence of AA and without light has been observed. [27,28] While PDT is limited to regions of the body accessible to light illumination, CT does not require light. Therefore CT is more flexible and adaptable for treatment of poorly accessible neoplasms. In cancer treatment, CT functions by various mechanisms including inducing direct cell death, damage to the tumor vasculature and stimulation of inflammation and nonspecific or specific immune effector cells. [29]

AA in cancer prevention

Breast Cancer: Plasma levels of AA were significantly lower while platelet levels were higher in a group of recently diagnosed breast cancer patients when compared to a matched group of controls. [30] Epidemiological studies appear to point to ascorbate as a possible chemopreventive for breast cancer. In the Iowa Women's Health Study, women who reported consuming at least 500mg AA daily showed a relative risk of developing breast cancer of 0.79 (not statistically significant) compared with women who did not supplement with AA. [31] Rohan et al., reported a small, statistically insignificant decrease in risks with AA consumption (as assessed by dietary reporting). [32] In a Spanish study comparing AA intake among breast cancer patients and matched controls, the cancer patients reported significantly lower intakes of dietary AA than controls. [33]

A meta-analysis of 12 studies and a number of different nutrients and their relationship to breast cancer found *AA intake has the most consistent and statistically significant inverse association with breast cancer risk.* [34] Verhoeven et al. found no significant association between AA supplementation and decreased breast cancer risk. To make the claim as they did however, that supplementation with AA does not confer protection from breast cancer is erroneous since their "higher doses" were an average of 165.3 mg daily. The group was divided according to supplemental intake as reported on a questionnaire into quintiles with the average reported intake of AA daily ranged from 58.6 mg in the lowest quintile to 165.3 mg in the highest). [35]

Cervical Cancer: A Latin American study compared nutrient intake and dietary patterns of 748 cervical cancer patients with 1,411 controls. The result supported a protective affect of AA against invasive cervical cancer. Other researchers have found a similar inverse relationship between cervical neoplasia and dietary AA. [36,37] A review article examining a number of studies concluded that in many but not all studies, an inverse relationship between AA status and the risk for cervical dysplasia was observed. [38]

Colorectal Cancer: Colonic polyps are recognized as a frequent precursor to colorectal cancer. In a group of 36 patients with polyps, 19 received 3 grams AA daily and 17 received placebo. The researchers noted a decrease in polyp area after nine months of treatment with AA but not with the placebo. In addition, a trend toward a decrease in polyp number was noted. Other researchers have used antioxidants to prevent recurrence of polyps in patients who had undergone surgical removal of their polyps. Patients were divided into three groups receiving either lactulose, a combination of vitamins A, C, and E, or nothing. Among 209 patients, polyps recurred in 5.7 percent of those given the vitamins, in 14.7 percent of those receiving lactulose and in 35.9 percent of the untreated control. [39]

An Australian study examining dietary habits and incidence of colorectal cancer found AA but not vitamin A to be protective. A similar study on patients of a major health plan in Los Angeles found a weak inverse relationship between supplemental and dietary AA and incidence of colorectal cancer. [40]

Cancer cells are the result of multiple genetic defects resulting from exposure to environmental, dietary and infectious agents. The dietary carcinogens such as N-nitroso compounds, polycyclic aromatic hydrocarbons and heterocyclic amines are present in cured or spoiled foods and crude oil contaminated diets. The level of exposure of cellular DNA to these and other carcinogens depends largely on the general quality of diet, the presence of bioactivated dietary constituents including antioxidant vitamins found in abundance in fruits and vegetables. In addition, normal cellular metabolizing enzymes convert particular chemicals to more water soluble compounds that can be excreted in the urine. [41]

Oxidative stress induction by crude oil was indicated by an increase in lipid peroxidation and a decrease in superoxide dismutase and catalase activities. However, pre-treatment of the diet with AA and vitamin E exhibited a protective role on the toxic effects of crude oil. The order of protection was vitamin E + C > vitamin E > vitamin C. [42]

Humans are readily exposed to preformed N-nitroso compounds (NOCs) and endogenous NOCs. Several NOCs are potential human carcinogens including N-nitrosodimethylamine (NDMA). There was a significant interaction between plasma AA concentration and dietary NDMA intake on cancer incidence. Plasma AA may modify the relation between NDMA exposure and cancer risk. [43]

References

[1] Lee JY, Chang MY, Park CH, Kim HY, Kim JH, Son H, Lee YS, Lee SH. Ascorbate induced differentiation of embryonic cortical precursors into neurons and astrocytes. Journal of Neuroscience Research 2003, 73(2), 156-165.

[2] Gonzalez MJ, Miranda-Massari JR, Mora EM, Guzmán A, Riordan NH, Riordan HD, Casciari JJ, Jackson JA, Román-Franco A. Orthomolecular Oncology Reviews: Ascorbic acid and cancer 25 years later. Integrative Cancer Therapies 2005, 4(1), 32.

[3] Mahdavi R, Faramarzi E, Seyedrezazadeh E, Mohammad-Zadeh M, Pourmoghaddam M.: Evaluation of oxidative stress, antioxidant status and cerum vitamin C levels in cancer patients. Biological Trace Element Research 2009, 130, 1-6.

[4] Pathak AK, Bhutani M, Guleria R, Bal S, Mohan A, Mohanti BK, Sharma A, Pathak R, Bhardwaj NK, Prasad KN, Kochupillai V. Chemotherapy alone vs. chemotherapy plus high dose multiple antioxidants in patients with advanced non small cell lung cancer. Journal of the American College of. Nutrition 2005, 24, 16-21.

[5] Fei B, Lawson S. Vitamin C and cancer revisited. Proceedings of the National Academy of Sciences of the USA 2008, 105, 11037-11038.

[6] Cameron E, Pauling L. Supplemental ascorbate in the supportive treatment of cancer: Revaluation of prolongation of survival times in terminal human cancer. Proceedings of the National Academiy of Sciences. USA 1978, 75, 4538-4532.

[7] Padayatty SJ, Riordan HD, Hewitt SM, Katz A, Hoffer LJ, Levine M. Intravenously administered vitamin C as cancer therapy: Three cases. Canadian Medical Association Journal 2006, 174, 937-942.

[8]   Roomi MW, Ivanov V, Kalinovsky T, Niedzwiecki A, Rath M. Antitumor effect of ascorbic acid, lysine, praline, arginine, and green tea extract on bladder cancer cell line T-24. International Journal of Urology, 2006, 13(4), 415-419.

[9]   Roomi MW, Ivanov V, Kalinovsky T, Niedzwiecki A, Rath M. Anticancer effect of lysine, praline, arginine, ascorbic acid and green tea extract on human renal adenocarcinoma line 786-0. Oncology Reports 2006, 16(5) 943-947.

[10]   Roomi MW, Kalinovsky T, Roomi NW, Monterrery J, Rath M, Niedzwiecki A. A nutrient mixture suppresses hepatic metastasis in athymic and mice injected with murine B16FO melanoma cells. Biofactors 2008, 33, 181-189.

[11]   Niedzwiecki A, Roomi MW, Kalinovsky T, Rath M. Micronutrient synergy—a new tool in effective control of metastasis and other key mechanisms of cancer. Cancer Metastasis Reviews. 2010, 29, 529-542.

[12]   Ichim TE, Minev B, Braciak T, Luna B, Hunninghake R, Mikirova NA, Jackson JA, Gonzalez MJ, Miranda-Massari JR, Alexandrescu DT, Dasanu CA, Bogin V, Ancans J, Stevens RB, Markosian B, Koropatnick J, Chen CS, Riordan NH. Intravenous ascorbic acid to prevent and treat cancer-associated sepsis. Journal of Translational Medicine 2011, 9, 25-38.

[13]   Gilloteaux J, Jacques G, Henryk ST, James MJ, Summers JL. Nontoxic potentiation sensitization of ovarian cancer therapy by supplementary treatment with vitamins US Patent 2007/0043110 Al. (22 Feb. 2007)

[14]   K. Plaetzer, T. Kiesslich, C.B. Oberdanner, B. Krammer: Apoptosis following photodynamic tumor therapy: induction, mechanisms and detection, Current Pharmaceutical Design 2005, 11, 1151-1165.

[15]   Fuchs J, Weber S, Kaufmann R. Genotoxic potential of porphyrin type photosensitizers with particular emphasis on 5-aminolevulinic acid: implications for clinical photodynamic therapy, Free Radical Biology & Medicine 2000, 28, 537-548.

[16]   Heck DE, Vetrano AM, Mariano TM, Laskin JD. UVB light stimulates production of reactive oxygen species: unexpected

role for catalase, Journal of Biological Chemistry 2003, 278, 22432-22436.

[17]   Heck DE, Gerecke DR, Vetrano AM, Laskin JD. Solar ultraviolet radiation as a trigger of cell signal transduction, toxicol. Applied Pharmacology 2004, 195, 288-297.

[18]   Vol'pin ME, Yu N, Krainova, I. Ya. Levitin IY.: B12 compounds in combination with ascorbic acid as potential antitumor agents, Mendeleev Chemistry Journal 1998, 42, 116-127.

[19]   Dikalov SI, Vitek MP, Mason RP. Cupricamyloid beta peptide complex stimulates oxidation of ascorbate and generation of hydroxyl radical, Free Radical Biology & Medicine 2004, 36, 340-347.

[20]   Akatov VS, Evtodienko YV, Leshchenko VV, Leshchenko VV, Teplova VV, Potselueva MM, Kruglov AG, Lezhnev EI, Yakubovskaya RI. Combined vitamins B12 and C induce the glutathione depletion and the death of epidermoid human larynx carcinoma cells HEp-2. Bioscience Reports 2000, 20, 411-418.

[21]   Proteggente AR, England TG, Rice-Evans CA: Iron supplementation and oxidative damage to DNA in healthy individuals with high plasma ascorbate. Biochemical Biophysical Research Communications 2001, 19, 245-251.

[22]   Proteggente AR, Rehman A, Halliwell B, Rice-Evans CA. Potential problems of ascorbate and iron supplementation: Pro-oxidant effect in vivo. Biochemical Biophysical Research Communications 2000, 277, 535-540.

[23]   Mikhailova LM, Ermakova NP, Chlenova EL. Toxicity of binary "theraphthal-Lio+ascorbic acid" (TPH+AA) catalytic system during different methods of regional intra-arterial administration in doges, Voprosy Onkologii 2001, 47, 710-714.

[24]   Mikhailova LM, Ermakova NP, Chlenova, EL. Preclinical toxicological study of theraphthal-Lio and binary catalytic system "theraphthal-Lio+ascorbic acid", Voprosy Onkologii 2001 47, 695-700.

[25]   Garin AM, Gorbunova VA, Gershanovich ML, Manziuk L.V, Borodkina AG, Breder VV, Karmanovskaia OB, Zubrikhina GN, Madzhuga AV, Zimakova NI, Trapeznikov NN. Results of a phase

I clinical trial of "theraphthal+ascorbic acid" catalytic system, Voprosy Onkologii 2001, 47, 676-700.

[26] Chen Q, Espey MG, Krishna MC, Mitchell JB, Corpe CP, Buettner GR, Shacter E, Levine M. Pharmacologic ascorbic acid concentrations selectively kill cancer cells: action as a pro-drug to deliver hydrogen peroxide to tissues, Proeedings of the National Academy of Sciences of the USA 2005, 102, 13604-13609.

[27] Magda D, Leep C, Gerasimchuk N, Lee I, Sessler JL, Lin A, Biaglow JE, Miller RA. Redox cycling by motexafin gadolinium enhances cellular response to ionizing radiation by forming reactive oxygen species. International Journal of Radiation Oncology Biology Physics 2001, 51, 1025-1036.

[28] Sessler JL and Miller RA. Texaphyrins: New drugs with diverse clinical application in radiation and photodynamic therapy, Biochemical Pharmacology 2000, 59, 733-739.

[29] Sharman ws, Allen CM, van Lier JE. Photodynamic therapeutics: basic principles and clinical applications, Drug Discovery Today 1999, 4(11), 507-517.

[30] Nunez MC, de Apodaca y Ruiz AO. Ascorbic acid in the plasma and blood cells of women with breast cancer. The effect of the consumption of food with an elevated content of this vitamin. Nutrición Hospitalaria 1995, 10, 368-372.

[31] Kishi LH, Fee RM, Sellers TA. Kushi LH, Fee RM, Sellers TA, Zheng W, Folsom AR. Intake of vitamins A. C and E and postmenopausal breast cancer. The Iowa Women's Health Study. American Journal of Epidemiology 1996, 144, 165-174.

[32] Rohan TE, Howe GR, Friedenreich CM, Jain M, Miller AB. Dietary fiber, vitamins A, C and E, and risk of breast cancer: a cohort study. Cancer Causes & Control 1993, 4, 29-37.

[33] Landa MC, Frago N, Tres A. Diet and the risk of breast cancer in Spain. European Journal of Cancer Prevention 1994, 3, 313-320.

[34] Block G. Vitamin C and cancer prevention: the epidemiological evidence. American Journal of Clinical Nutrition 1991, 53, 270S-282S.

[35] Verhoeven DTH, Assen N, Goldbohm RA, Dorant E, van 't Veer P, Sturmans F, Hermus RJ, van den Brandt PA. Vitamins C and E,

retinol, beta-carotene and dietary fibre in relation to breast cancer risk: a prospective cohort study. British Journal of Cancer 1997, 75, 149-155.

[36] VanEenwyk J, Davis FG, Colman N. Folate, vitamin C, and cervical intraepithelial neoplasia. Cancer Epidemiology, Biomarkers & Prevention 1992, 1, 119-124.

[37] Liu T, Soong SJ, Wilson NP, Craig CB, Cole P, Macaluso M, Butterworth CE. A case control study of nutritional factors and cervical dysplasia. Cancer Epidemiology, Biomarkers and Prevention 1993, 2, 525-530.

[38] Potischman N, Brinton L. Nutrition and cervical neoplasia. Cancer Causes & Control, 1996, 7, 113-126.

[39] Ponz de Leon M, Roncucci L. Chemoprevention of colorectal tumors: role of lactulose and of other agents. Scandanavian Journal of Gastroenterology, Supplement 1997, 222, 72-75.

[40] Enger SM, Longnecker MP, Chen MJ, Harper J.M., Lee E.R., Frankl H.D., Haile R.W. Dietary intake of specific carotenoids and vitamins A. C and E, and prevalence of colorectal adenomas. Cancer Epidemiology, Biomarkers and Prevention 1996, 5, 147-153.

[41] Herber B and Go VLW. Future directions in cancer and nutrition research: gene-nutrient interaction and the xenobiotic hypothesis. In: Nutrition/Oncology pp. 613-618 Academic Press, San Diego, CA. (1999).

[42] Fidelis I, Achuba, EOO. Protective influence of vitamins against petroleum-induced free radical toxicity in rabbit. Environmentalist 2006, 26, 295-300.

[43] N-Nitroso compounds and cancer incidence: the European Prospective Investigation into Cancer and Nutrition (EPIC)-Norfolk Study. American Journal of Clinical Nutrition 2011, 93(5), 1053-61.

Nanotechnology and Cancer Prevention, Detection and Treatment

Dr Nadia G. Kandile

Professor of Applied Chemistry,
Department of Chemistry,
Faculty of Women, Ain Shams University,
Heliopolis, 1175, Cairo, Egypt

Abstract

This chapter is an overview of the advances and prospects for the application of nanotechnology for cancer prevention, detection and treatment. A brief description of cancer is followed by a brief discussion of nanoparticle science as the foundation upon which most nanotechnology cancer therapy is based. Nanotechnology is shown to be an important component in the challenging quest to solve this affliction which is one of the most challenging and longstanding problems in medicine.

Introduction

Cancer remains one of the most complex diseases affecting humans and despite the impressive advances that have been made in molecular and cell biology, cancer cell progression through to carcinogenesis and the subsequent acquisition of metastatic ability is still widely debated. The idea that cancer might be attributed to inherent changes within the organism's own genome did not arise until after the discovery that retroviruses could transform host cells. Often the host_cells contain variants of cellular genes which are necessary for oncogenic transformation. Consequently for perhaps nearly twenty years, the field of oncology was synonymous with virology and a major focus was on identifying these proto-oncogenes or genes that could be turned into cancer-causing genes. Today, cancer is recognized as a highly heterogeneous disease and over 100 distinct types have been described with various tumor subtypes found within specific organs. It is now also recognized that genetic and phenotypical variabilities primarily determine the self-progressive growth, invasiveness and metastatic potential of neoplastic disease and its response or resistance to therapy. It seems that this multilevel complexity of cancer explains the clinical diversity of histologically similar neoplasias.

Recent advances in other disciplines have uncovered that in addition to viral infection, disregulation of many normal cellular processes such as gene regulation, cell cycle control, DNA repair and replication, checkpoint signaling, differentiation and apoptosis can lead to cancer. The mechanisms of transformation can be complex with multiple pathways affected. [1]

In addition to multiple pathways being compromised in tumor cells, tumors can arise in a cell or tissue specific manner. For instance, mutations in the breast cancer susceptibility gene, *BRCA1* are associated with approximately half of the inherited forms of breast and ovarian cancer but they do not predispose carriers to most other forms of cancer even though the gene is ubiquitously expressed and is involved in the fundamental processes of transcriptional regulation and DNA repair. [2].

While sometimes there are common mutations frequently associated with many cancers, the majority of cancers arise from a diverse array of malfunctions that result in a tumor that is unique to that patient. The complexity of cancer combined with an avalanche of basic scientific research uncovers a plethora of pathways that feed into cellular growth control reveals many potential therapeutic targets. As such, there is a critical need for cancer biologists with a broad knowledge of the mechanisms of tumorigenesis to team up with clinical oncologists to address just how this information can be utilized to advance clinical therapies.

The National Cancer Institute (NCI), USA has recognized these critical clinical deficiencies and has been on the forefront of identifying and developing new and innovative ways to approach cancer diagnosis, treatment and management. Having witnessed substantial technological advances in the field of nanotechnology in various disciplines including physical sciences, engineering, physics and chemistry in developing new materials and devices to be used in electronics and energy conservation, the NCI recognizes nanotechnology as an exciting and promising approach to address cancer applications as well.

Nanotechnology is the study and application of matter at atomic and molecular levels. More specifically, nanotechnology involves substances that are nanoscale, that is, the matter has at least one dimension between 1 and 100 nanometres (one nanometre is a billionth of a metre) as shown in **Figure 1**.

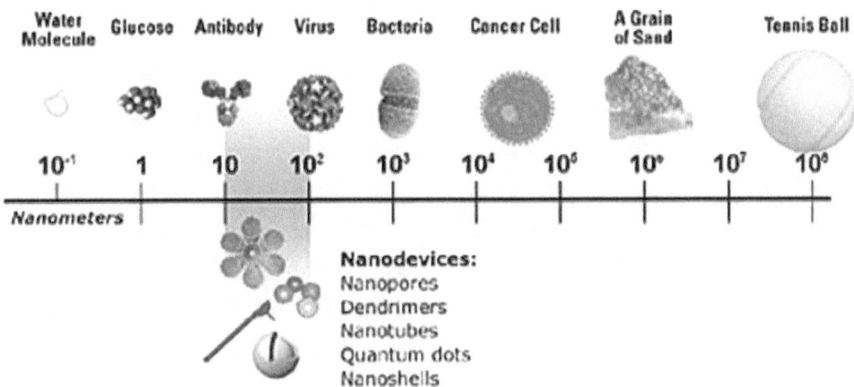

Figure 1. Relative size of a nanometer.
Source http://www.tacc.utexas.edu/research/users/features/ nano.php

The arrival of nanotechnology enabled engineers to construct materials from the "bottom up" as opposed to making a current machine or a structure dramatically smaller. It was in the early 1980s that nanotechnology had its first two developments: the arrival of cluster science and the creation of the scanning tunneling microscope as depicted in **Figure 2**.

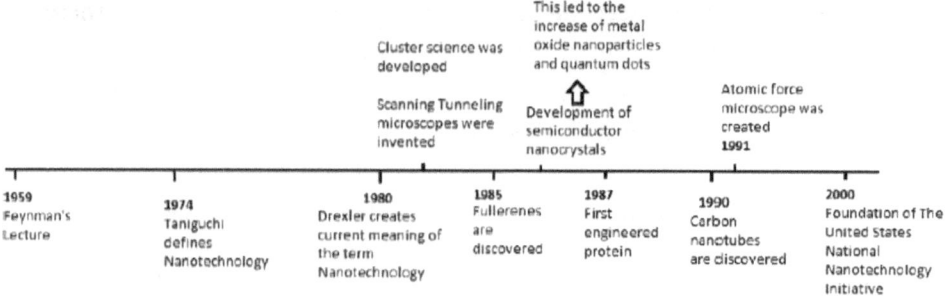

Figure 2. History of nanotechnology.

Nanotechnology involves research and technology development at the atomic, molecular or macromolecular levels and allows the creation and use of functionalized structures, devices and systems that take advantage of specific properties of matter that exist at the nanoscale. Nanoscale structures can be manipulated on the atomic scale and integrated into larger material components, systems and architectures. The potential for using nanotechnology in medicine and especially in the area of cancer is vast. For example, nanoparticles targeting tumor cells, using the knowledge we have about cellular biology will enable clinicians to deliver therapy specifically to the tumor while reducing unwanted side effects. In addition, increased capacity to image tumor cells will enable earlier diagnosis, confer increased accuracy for surgical resection, offer real-time assessment of treatment effectiveness and enhance monitoring for metastasis or primary tumor re-growth. Furthermore, powerful chemotherapeutic agents that have been abandoned due to toxic side effects can be resurrected using nanotechnology enabled delivery systems thus allowing them to become viable treatment options. Cancer is a complex disease occurring as a result of a progressive accumulation of genetic and epigenetic changes that enable escape from normal cellular and environmental control [3].

Cancer is a generic term for a group of more than 100 diseases that can affect any part of the body. Other terms used are malignant tumors (severe and progressively worsening tumors) and neoplasms (abnormal masses of tissue resulting from abnormal proliferation of cells). One defining feature of cancer is the rapid creation of abnormal cells which grow beyond their usual boundaries and which can invade adjoining parts of the body and spread to other organs: a process referred to as metastasis. Metastases are the major cause of death from cancer. [4]

The field of nanotechnology was first predicated by Professor Richard P Feynman in 1959 (Nobel laureate in physics, 1965) with his famous Cal Tech Lecture entitled, ***There's plenty of room at the bottom***. [5]

Recently, functional nanoparticles have been developed that are covalently linked to biological molecules such as peptides, proteins, nucleic acids or small molecule ligands. [6-14]

Medical applications have also appeared, such as the use of super paramagnetic iron oxide nanoparticles as a contrast agent for lymph node prostate cancer detection. [14]

Nanotechnology preventive medicine approach

In general, the best way to eliminate a problem is to eliminate the cause. In cancer, the problem can be perceived differently at various stages of the disease. Most apparent, if genetic mutations are the underlying cause, then we must counteract the causes of the mutations. Unfortunately, genetic mutations are caused by artificial or natural carcinogens only some of the time. At other times, they may occur spontaneously during DNA replication and cell division. With the present state of science and technology, there is very little we can do to prevent this from happening. However, in all other cases eliminating the carcinogens is indeed a highly effective way of cancer prevention. But most patients do not recognize the problem until it has actually occurred. This fact means preventive medicine a rarely utilized, even though a highly effective form of cancer prevention. Even so, is there a way to eliminate cancer through nanotechnology before it starts? Although there is little current research on preventive treatments using nanotechnology, nanotechnology is indeed possible and indeed holds much promise at this time. After a careful review of the most advanced disease-time nanoscale treatment methods, one can easily see why the proposed nanotechnology alternatives to current preventive treatments have so strongly attracted the attention of the scientific and medical communities in recent years. In fact, nanotechnology-based treatments are no more challenging to devise than the currently used disease-time treatment methods. Nonetheless, it requires time and monetary investments to develop such treatment methods in a short period of time.

To demonstrate the viability of the nanotechnology based treatments, let us consider melanoma as an example. Melanoma, a form of skin cancer is caused primarily by ultraviolet radiation from the sun as indicated in **Figure 3**. The current method of preventive treatment against bombardment with this kind of harmful radiation involves suspending a substance that either absorbs or scatters ultraviolet radiation in a thick emulsion. We use emulsions called sunscreens to coat our skin prior to prolonged exposure to sunlight.

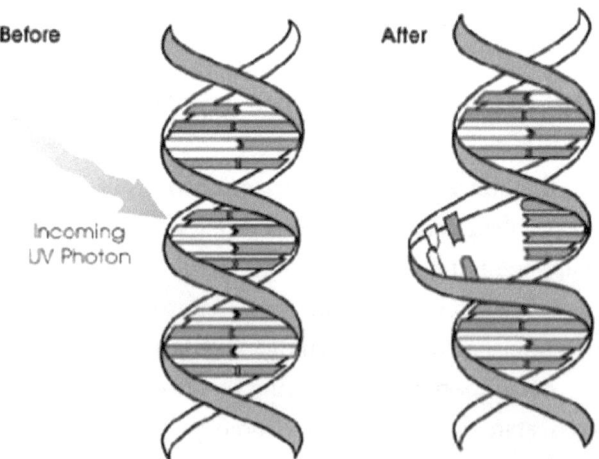

Figure 3. UV damage of DNA. UV radiation is one of the most prominent causes of DNA damage. Since UV radiation is high frequency and thus high energy, it can easily damage the delicate DNA double helix. Individual nucleotide bases readily absorb UV radiation and can easily become excited even after short term

exposure. This can cause hydrogen bonds between two complimentary chains, and sometimes even the covalent bonds between the phosphate backbone and the ribose to break, causing genetic mutants. The result a mutated genetic sequence and the production of defective proteins.

Source: http://earthobservatory.nasa.gov/ Library/UVB/Images/dna_mutation.gif

Some very recent studies have shown that it is possible to tag specific types of cells with nanoparticles by conjugating them to targeting agents designed to recognize cell specific surface proteins. [16] Nanoparticles attached to desired drugs or substances can be conjugated to short peptide chains, proteins or artificial nanobodies. Nanoparticles can be prepared attached to UV scattering substances like zinc oxide (ZnO) and titanium oxide (TiO_2) or UV absorbing substances like octyl methoxycinnamate and oxybenzone **Figure 4**. These modified nanoparticles can then specifically target skin cell surface proteins. The skin cells are thus effectively coated with sunscreen on the nanoscale. With this nanotechnology based preventive treatment, many of the above problems can be effectively eliminated. If the cells can be coated directly, the problem of diffraction in cases were an area, even if sparsely coated will be eliminated. The most important issue to consider in this form of treatment is of course, the toxicity of the substance that is used. The biochemical effects of a substance on the patient's health must be thoroughly evaluated by standard laboratory testing procedures as well as clinical trials before this treatment can be safely implemented. Of course, this is a purely theoretical suggestion, which is based on what are unrelated to skin cells.

Figure 4. Two examples of ultraviolet radiation absorbing organic substances. a. octyl methoxycinnamate, b. oxybenzone

The sunscreen issue is proposed simply as an example of a single potential application of nanotechnology. However, if this method can indeed be turned into reality, the obvious result will be a large reduction in the incident of melanoma due to the sun's radiation. Some of the problems with this method are that the emulsion can be easily rubbed off and can lose its effectiveness over time, thus needing reapplication periodically. An even bigger problem is that openings are left in the sunscreen coating during application due to macroscale and microscale imperfections in our skin. This allows the ultraviolet (UV) radiation to permeate through the dead layer of skin, spreading out to a wider area due to slit diffraction and then cause more widespread damage. All of these problems detract from the overall effectiveness of this preventive method.

It is possible to quickly and easily map large proteins and model them in three-dimensional space [17] as well as obtain extensive knowledge of atomic and molecular interactions [18] and electronic cloud distributions. [19] It is also possible to sequence and manufacture nucleic acid and peptide chains readily. [20] Taken all together, these techniques give us all that we need in order to specifically target any type of animal cell provided that it can be distinguished from other cell types by the presence of at least one cell-specific surface protein. Thus, the method discussed above is but one example of many possible applications of the fascinating new nanotechnology known as nanobiotechnology.

Engineered nanoparticles have the potential to revolutionize the diagnosis and treatment of many diseases; for example, by allowing the targeted delivery of a drug to particular subsets of cells. However, so far such nanoparticles have not proven capable of surmounting all of the biological barriers required to achieve this goal. Nevertheless, advances in nanoparticle engineering, as well as the understanding of the importance of nanoparticle characteristics such as size, shape and surface properties for biological interactions have created new opportunities for the development of nanoparticles for therapeutic applications. In the past two decades, several therapeutics based on nanoparticles have been successfully introduced for the treatment of cancer, pain and infectious diseases. [21-23]

This type of therapeutic harnesses the opportunities provided by nanomaterials to target the delivery of drugs more specifically, improve solubility, extend half-life, improve therapeutic index, allow controlled release and reduce immunogenicity.

The concept of chemoprevention gained momentum when numerous laboratory studies showed anticancer effects of natural agents in various tumor models. [24] However, natural agents failed to prove their worth at the last and most expensive step, i.e. in the clinic. [25] Many reasons have been attributed to this failure. These range from lack of a clearly defined mechanism of action to poor bioavailability. [26] Further, the observed anticancer activity of different natural agents in cell culture and animal models does not translate into clinically beneficial outcomes in humans. This is because laboratory studies tend to investigate pharmacological effects at doses that are not achievable in humans through dietary sources. [27] Based on these important and limiting factors, the science of chemoprevention has fewer proponents and more critics. Nevertheless since, the term chemoprevention was coined 40 years ago [28,29] researchers through extensive high throughput screening have identified an arsenal of anticancer drugs from natural sources. [30] The natural agent fleet is led by the flagship drug Taxol which has been approved by the FDA for the treatment of several human malignancies. [31] Many other drugs, originally discovered from nature have also been approved by the FDA, including camptothecin and its analogs (topotecan and irinotecan), vinblastine and vincristine and the anthracyclines (from microbial sources) such as doxorubicin and the bleomycins [32-36]. Several other promising compounds are currently being tested in clinical trials against cancer and other deadly chronic diseases.

Compounds such as resveratrol [37-39], curcumin [40,41], thymoquinone [42-44] and epigallocatechin (EGCG) have shown potent anticancer activity in cell culture and animal tumor models [45-51]. These chemopreventive agents have also demonstrated some clinical benefit in combination with standard chemotherapeutics—the synergistic effect.

However, despite promising results in preclinical settings, the applicability of these agents to humans has met with only limited success, largely due to inefficient systemic delivery and bioavailability. For example, the study of pharmacokinetics of resveratrol in humans concluded that even high doses of resveratrol might be insufficient to achieve resveratrol concentrations required for the systemic prevention of cancer. [52] Similarly, the amount of EGCG or curcumin required to observe anticancer effects in humans is too high to be feasibly incorporated in a clinical trial due to acute toxicity. [53] Therefore, to achieve the maximum response of a chemopreventive agent, novel strategies are required to enhance the bioavailability of potentially useful agents and reduce perceived toxicity.

Nanomedical approaches to drug delivery center on developing nanoscale particles or molecules to improve drug bioavailability. [54,55] Drug delivery focuses on maximizing bioavailability both at specific places in the body and over a period of time. Numerous different strategies have been employed in nanotechnology to optimize drug delivery in a tumor specific manner. This technology extends to different disciplines of science such as chemistry, environmental science, tissue engineering as well as in medicine where it is gradually cementing its position as a potent therapeutic option. Different approaches have been applied to effectively load target drugs to enhance delivery that are based on the solubility properties of drugs to be loaded as discussed below.

Nanotechnology and cancer detection

The theme of nanotechnology is the control of material on a scale of 1 to 100 nanometers and fabricates the devices on this scale of length. On the nano scale, there is a vast increase in the ratio of surface area to volume to anything bigger. Due to this, materials at the nanoscale show very different properties compared to those they exhibit on a micro scale, enabling unique applications. [56] For instance:

- opaque substances become transparent (example copper)
- inert materials becomes catalysts (example platinum)
- stable materials become combustible (example aluminium)
- solids turn into liquids at room temperature (example gold)
- insulators become conductors (example silicon).

A material such as gold which is inert can become a potent chemical catalyst at the nanoscale. Some of the unique applications of nanomaterials include

- titanium dioxide nanoparticles in sunscreens
- cosmetics and some food products
- silver nanoparticles in food packing, clothing, disinfectants and household appliances
- zinc oxide nanoparticles in cosmetics, surface coatings, paints and outdoor furniture varnishes.

However, further applications that require actual manipulations or arrangement of nanoscale components await further research.

Nanotechnology has the potential to produce a revolutionary impact on cancer diagnosis and therapy. It is universally accepted that early detection of cancer is essential, even before anatomic anomalies are visible. A major challenge in cancer diagnosis in the 21st century is to be able to determine the exact relationship between cancer biomarkers and the clinical pathology, as well as be able to non-invasively detect tumors at an early stage for maximum therapeutic benefit. For breast cancer for instance, the goal of molecular imaging is to be able to accurately diagnose when the tumor mass contains approximately 100-1000 cells, as opposed to the current techniques like mammography, which require more than a million cells for accurate clinical diagnosis.

Cancer detection—conventional detection

Conventional detection of the cancer is done by observing the physical growth/changes in the organ by X-ray and/or CT scanning and is confirmed by biopsy through cell culture. However the limitation of this method is that it is not very sensitive and the detection is possible only after substantial growth of the cancerous cells. Often the treatment is also not possible once the cancer is in such an advanced stage.

Cancer detection—nanotechnology detection

As mentioned before, nanoparticles (NP) are of a few of nanometres and the cells are of the size of few microns. So NP can enter into the cells and can access the DNA and hence affect genes. There is a possibility that the defect in the genes can be detected. DNA molecules can be detected in their incipient stage. This could be possible *in vivo* or *in vitro*. It will be shown later that nanoparticles do show potential for cancer detection in its incipient stage.

Nanotechnology in cancer therapy

Some nanotechnology tools have applications in cancer detection and treatment and are discussed as follows:

(i) **Cantilevers:** Cantilevers are tiny bars anchored at one end and can be engineered to bind at the other end to molecules associated with cancer. These molecules may bind to DNA altered proteins that are present in certain types of cancer and are shown in **Figure 5**. This will change the surface tension and cause the cantilevers to bend. By monitoring the bending of cantilevers, it would be possible to tell whether the cancer molecules are present and hence detect early molecular events in the development of cancer.

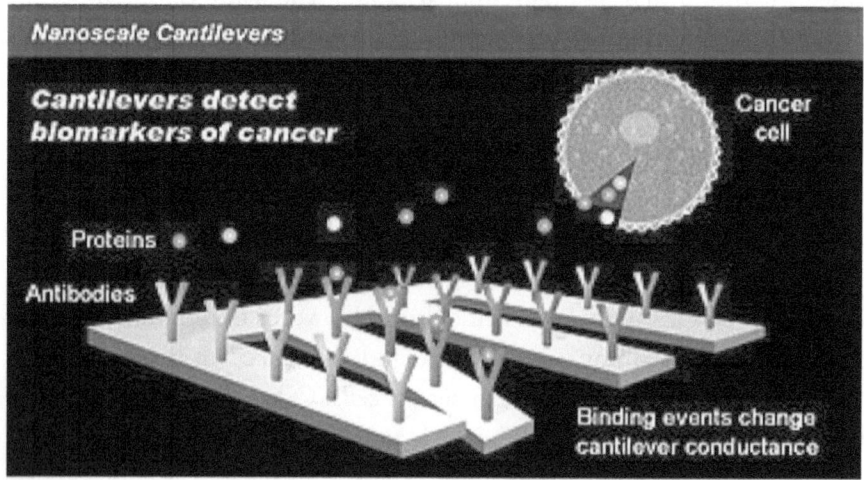

Figure 5. Schematic diagram showing cantilevers.
Source: National Cancer Institute, USA.

(ii)   Nanopores: Nanopores (holes) allow DNA to pass through one strand at a time and hence DNA sequencing can be made more efficient. Thus the shape and electrical properties of each base on the strand can be monitored. As these properties are unique for each of the four bases that make up the genetic code, the passage of DNA through a nanopore can be used to decipher the encoded information, including errors in the code known to be associated with cancer.

(iii) Nanotubes: Nanotubes are smaller than nanopores. Nanotubes and carbon rods are about half the diameter of a molecule of DNA. They will also help identify DNA changes associated with cancer Figure 6. Nanotubes help to exactly pinpoint the location of the changes. Mutated regions associated with cancer are first tagged with bulky molecules. Using a nanotube tip, resembling the needle on a record player, the physical shape of the DNA can be traced.

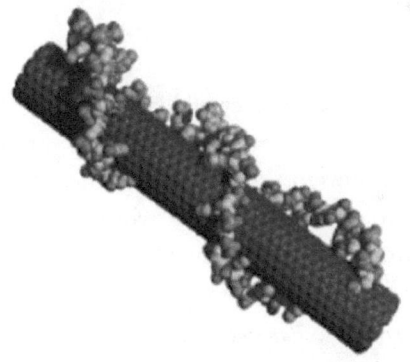

Figure 6. Schematics of a functionalised single-walled carbon nanotube with Cyanine Dye #3 labelled DNA (Cy3-DNA).

Source: Kam NWS, O'Connell M, Wisdom JA, Dai H. Carbon nanotubes as multifunctional biological transporters and near-infrared agents for selective cancer cell destruction. Proceedings of the National Academy of Sciences 2001, 102, 11600-11605.

A computer translates this information into topographical map. The bulky molecules identify the regions on the map where mutations are present. Since the location of mutations can influence the effects they have on a cell, these techniques will be important in predicting disease.

(iv)   Quantum Dotes (QD): These are tiny crystals that glow when they are stimulated by ultraviolet light. The latex beads filled with these crystals are stimulated by light. The colors they emit act as dyes that light up the sequence of interest. By combining different sized quantum dots within a single bead, probes can be created that release a distinct spectrum of various colors and intensities of lights, serving as spectral bar code Figure 7.

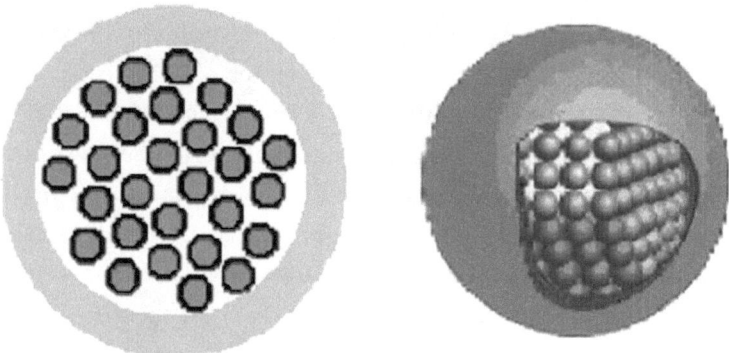

Figure 7. Semiconductor nanosize crystalline quantum dots possess quantised energy levels with unique optical and electronic properties. They confine electrons in three dimensions to a region, of the order of the electrons' de Broglie wavelength with varied sizes and shapes which can be precisely controlled containing anything from a single electron to a set of hundreds or even thousands of electrons.

Sources: Murray CB, Norris DJ, Bawendi MG. Synthesis and characterization of nearly monodisperse CdE (E = sulfur, selenium, tellurium) semiconductor nanocrystallites. Journal of the American Chemical Society 1993, 115, 8706-8715 and Gao X, Yang L, Petros JA, Marshall FE, Simons JW, Nie S. In vivo molecular and cellular imaging with quantum dots. Current Opinion in Biotechnology 2001. 16(1), 63-72.

(v)   Gold nanoparticles/nanoshells (NS): Gold nanoparticles/nanoshells (NS) are another recent invention. NS are miniscule beads coated with gold. By manipulating the thickness of the layers making up the NS, the beads can be designed to absorb a specific wavelength of light. The most useful nanoshells are those that absorb near infrared light that can easily penetrate several centimeters of human tissues. Absorption of light by nanoshells creates an intense heat that is lethal to cells. NS can be linked to antibodies that recognize cancer cells. In laboratory cultures, the heat generated by the light-absorbing nanoshells has successfully killed tumor cells while leaving neighboring cells intact.

(vi)   Dendrimer: A number of nanoparticles that will facilitate drug delivery are being developed. Dendrimers form a family of molecules that have the potential to link treatment with detection, diagnosis and therapy in a single molecule. These molecules have a have branching shape that gives them vast surface areas to which therapeutic agents or other biologically active molecules can be attached. A single dendrimer can carry a molecule that recognizes cancer cells, a molecule that recognizes the signals of cell death and a therapeutic agent to kill those cells. It is hoped that dendrimers can be manipulated to release their contents only in the presence of certain trigger molecules associated with cancer Figure 8(a,b).

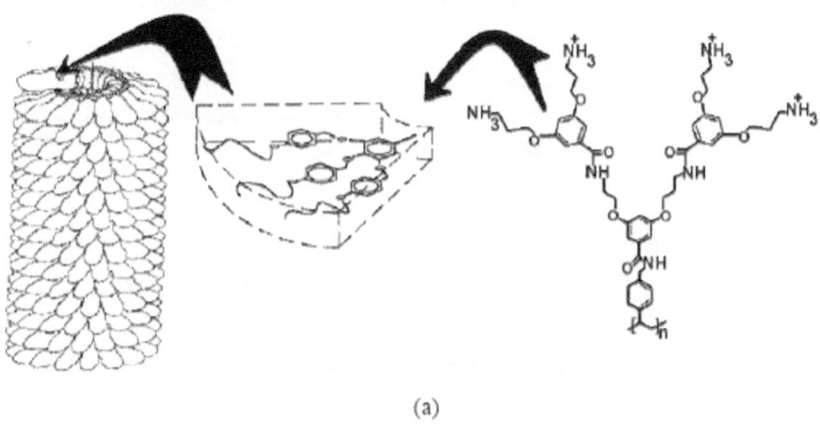

(a)

Figure 8(a). An example of a dendrimer used to carry a variety of agents fulfilling various functions. Shown here is the chemical structure and formation of a poly-amidoamine (PMAMA) dendrimer nanocylinder (dendronised polymer) which is used to carry a DNA molecule.

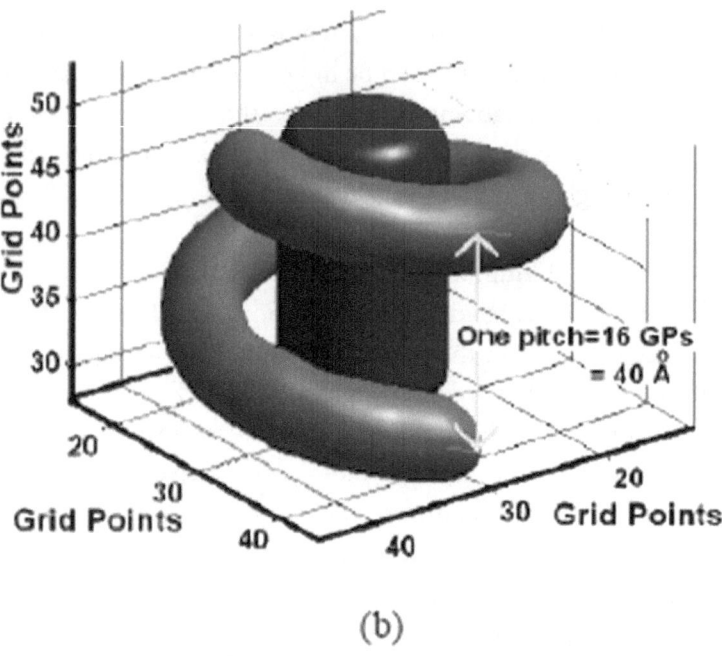

(b)

Figure 8(b). Format of DNA wrapped around the dendronised polymer resulting in 40Å pitch (single helix characterized by the height per turn).

Source: Nikakhtar A, Nasehzadeh A, Beidokhti HN, Mansoori GA. DNA-dendrimer nano-cluster electrostatics prediction with the non-linear Poission-Boltzman equation. Journal of Computational and Theoretical Nanoscience 2005, 2, 1-7.

(vii) **Liposomes:** Liposomes consist of synthetic microscopic fat globules of lipids which have a high level of highly biodegradability **Figure 9.** They are nanoscale closed vesicles consisting of a single lipid bilayer. They are manufactured to enclose medications for drug delivery for chemotherapy [57]. The fatty outer layer of the liposome confines and protects the enclosed drug until the liposome is delivered and adheres to the outer membrane of target cancer cells. By this process drug toxicity to healthy cells is decreased and its efficacy may be increased. Liposome therapy is a well-developed technology for delivery of chemotherapy drugs. [58-60]

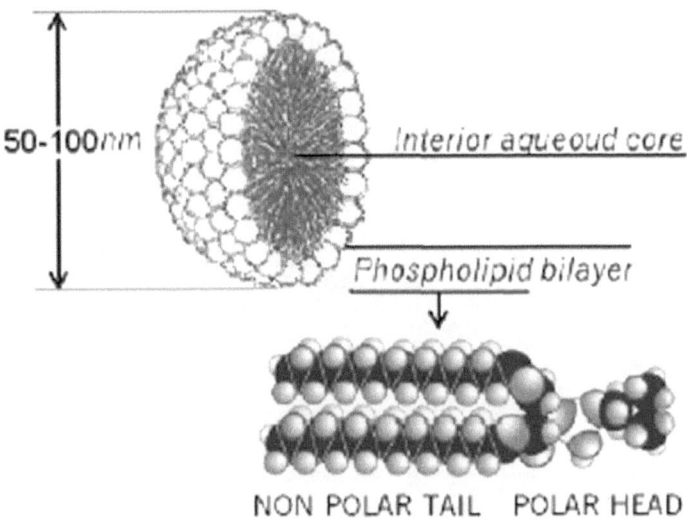

50-100nm   Interior aqueoud core

Phospholipid bilayer

NON POLAR TAIL   POLAR HEAD

Figure 9. Cross section of a liposome: a synthetic lipid bilayer vesicle that fuses with the outer cell membrane and is used to transport small molecules (example a drug) to tissues and into cells.

Source: Mansoori GA and and Soelaiman TAF. (2005) Principles of Nanotechnology: Molecular Based Study of Condensed Matter in Small Systems, World Scientific Pub. Co., New York.

(viii) Magnetic nanoparticles: Nanoscale magnetic particles with a variety of compositions, sizes and stabilisers have been prepared in the past four decades. Several applications for these materials exist, such as ferrofluids [61] in the solid state, primarily in the biomedical and magnetic recording industries. Magnetic nanoparticles were first discovered in a biological organism (chitons) in 1962. [62] Numerous current and potentially commercial biomedical applications exist for systems comprised of magnetic nanoparticles. Current applications are focused on *in vitro* applications such as cell and cell organelle detection and separation, immobilization, isolation and determination of biologically active compounds **Figure 10.**

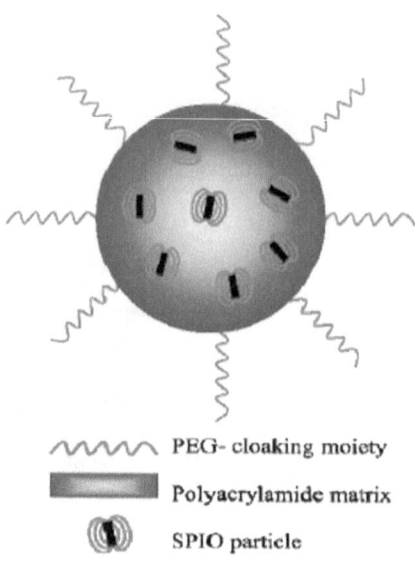

PEG- cloaking moiety

Polyacrylamide matrix

SPIO particle

Figure 10. Structure of a super paramagnetic iron oxide (SPIO) polyacrylamide magnetic (PAM) nanoparticle. SPIO paramagnetic characteristics have made them good candidates for *in vivo* cancer cell destruction through hyperthermia. Their polymer coating prevents their cytotoxicity and allows them to move freely in the organism without adhesion or reaction. Source: Moffat BA, Reddy GR, McConville P, Hall DE, Chenevert TL, Kopelman RR, Philbert M, Weissleder R, Rehemtulla A, Ross BD A novel polyacrylamiden magnetic nanoparticle contrast agent for molecular imaging using MRI. Molecular Imaging 2001 2(4), 324-332.

Nanomaterial biocompatibility. Predicting toxicology based on nanoparticle structure.

NCL-generated data has elucidated trends in nanomaterial characteristics and identified critical parameters that influence nanomaterial biocompatibility **Figure 11**. This data has contributed substantially to the current understanding of the *nanobio interface*. For example, particles must be smaller than approximately 200 nanometers to transverse the architecture of the liver and spleen. Particles that are hydrophobic (e.g. without a PEGylation layer) will quickly be removed from circulation by macrophages in the reticuloendothelial system (RES). With respect to elimination, particles and/or their breakdown products must be less than 10 nm to be excreted through the kidneys. Otherwise they may reside in the RES organs for the lifetime of the animal. However, particles as large as 30 nm may be excreted in the bile. Finally, cationic (strongly positively charged) particles are cytotoxic, with or without the chemotherapeutic agent onboard. Investigators should engineer particles with these parameters in mind and exploit the advantageous particle characteristics to hopefully avoid repeating the trial and error studies of the past.

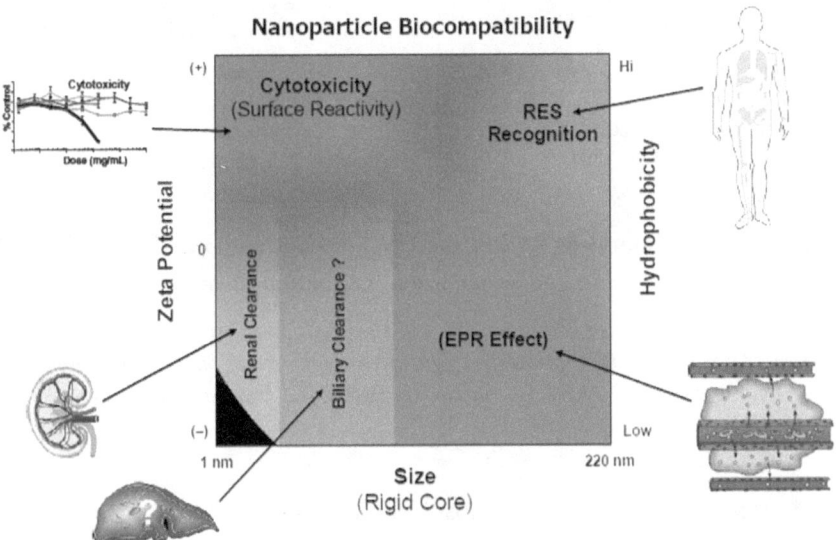

Figure 11. Nanoparticle biocompatibility. This plot shows trends the NCL has observed in the relationship between nanoparticle physico-chemical properties and biological responses. The independent variables in this plot are the zeta potential (related to surface charge), size and hydrophobicity which are plotted versus the dependent variable of biocompatibility. These variables are manifested in such biological responses as cytotoxicity, clearance, the EPR effect and RES recognition.

Source: McNeil SE. Nanoparticle therapeutics: a personal perspective. Wiley interdisciplinary reviews. Nanomedicine and nanobiotechnology 2009, 1, 264-271.

Types of Nano Formulations

The choice of nano formulation to be used depends on the solubility of the drug of interest that has to be loaded. The two most popular and well investigated drug carriers are liposomes (for the delivery of water soluble drugs) and micelles (for the delivery of water insoluble drugs) **Figure 12.**

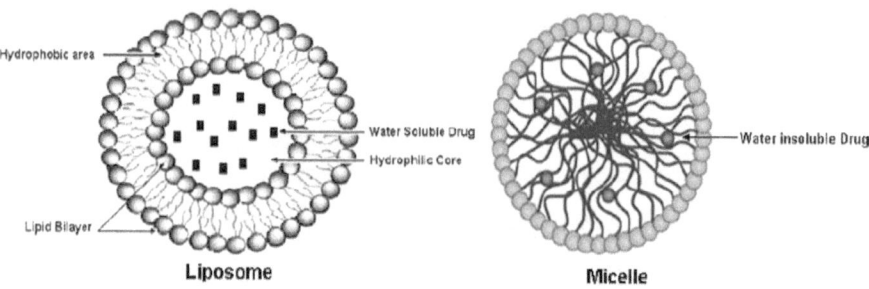

Figure 12. Two major drug loading models, liposome and micelle, for effectively loading of water soluble and water insoluble natural chemopreventive agents, respectively.

Source: *The micelle image is a modified figure from biomaterials for promoting protection, repair and regeneration. Orive G, Anitua E, Pedras JL, Emerich DL. Nature Reviews Neuroscience. 2009, 10, 682-692.*

Liposomes are artificial phospholipid vesicles that are usually less than 1,000 nm in size and can be loaded with a variety of water soluble drugs that sit in its inner compartment. Without doubt these liposomes have been considered to be promising drug carriers. [63,64] They are biologically inert and completely biocompatible and they cause practically no toxic or antigenic reactions. Drugs included in liposomes are protected from the destructive action of external media. [65] The use of targeted liposomes (that is liposomes selectively accumulating inside an affected organ or tissue) increases the efficacy of the liposomal drug and decreases the loss of liposomes and their contents in the reticuloendothelial system. [66,67] To obtain targeted liposomes, many protocols have been developed to bind corresponding targeting moieties, including antibodies, to the liposome surface without affecting the liposome integrity and antibody properties [68,69]. However, the approach with immunoliposomes may nevertheless be limited due to their short life in the circulation. [70,71]

Dramatically better accumulation can be achieved if the circulation time of liposomes is extended. This increases the total quantity of immunoliposomes passing through the target and increasing their interactions with target antigens. This is why long circulating (usually coated with PEG, i.e. PEGylated) liposomes have attracted so much attention over the last decade. [72]

The development of drug nanocarriers for water insoluble drugs has been a huge task, particularly because large proportions of new drug candidates emerging from high throughput drug screening initiatives such as chemopreventive agents that are water insoluble. The therapeutic application of hydrophobic, poorly water soluble agents such as curcumin, resveratroland and epigallocatechin gallate (EGCG) is associated with some serious problems, since low water solubility results in poor absorption and low bioavailability. [73] In addition, drug aggregation upon intravenous administration of poorly soluble drugs might lead to severe toxicity. On the other hand, hydrophobicity and low solubility water appear to be intrinsic properties of many drugs, since these characteristics help a drug molecule to penetrate the cell membrane and reach important intracellular targets. This is why micelles, including polymeric micelles are another promising type of pharmaceutical carrier for such water insoluble drugs. [74]

Micelles are colloidal dispersions with a particle size between 5 and 100 nm. An important property of micelles is their ability to increase the solubility and bioavailability of poorly soluble pharmaceuticals. The use of certain special amphiphilic molecules such as micelle building blocks can also extend the blood half-life upon intravenous administration. Because of their small size (<100 nm), micelles demonstrate spontaneous penetration into the body compartments with leaky vasculature. In the case of targeted micelles, local release of a free drug from micelles in the target organ should lead to increased efficacy of the drug, while the stability of the micelles *en route* to the target organ or tissue should contribute better drug solubility and toxicity reduction, because of less interaction with non-target organs.

Nanochemoprevention

The origin of nanoencapsulation based chemoprevention approaches can be traced to Mukhtar and co-workers who also coined the term nanochemoprevention for the first time. This group utilized the multi functionality of biodegradable polylactic acid (PLA)—polyethylene glycol (PLA-PEG) nanoparticles to incorporate the well recognized hemopreventive agent from green tea, EGCG. This revolutionary strategy showed effective antitumor efficacy in a prostate model and most importantly the PLA/PLGA [poly (DL-lactide-co-glycolide acid)] nanoparticles when injected systemically were rapidly cleared by the mononuclear phagocytic system by the process of endocytosis, thereby minimizing carrier induced undesirable cytotoxicity Figure 13. [75]

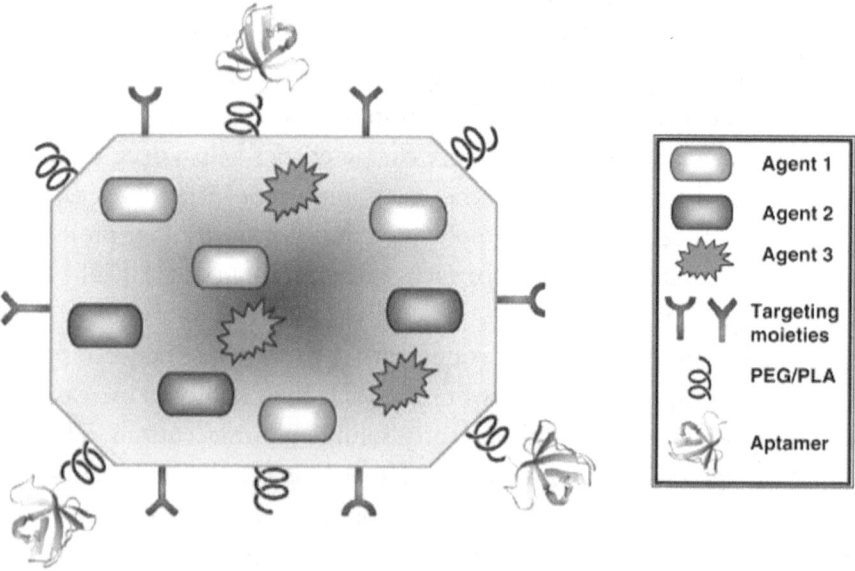

Figure 13. Multifunctional nanoparticles. The nanoparticles could be developed with an ability to carry one or more therapeutic agents. The surface of the nanoparticles could be conjugated to one or more targeting moieties, like antibodies or other recognition agents, and polyethylene glycol (PEG)/polylactic

acid (PLA) could be added for the avoidance of uptake by macrophages. The surface of the nanoparticles could also contain aptamers conjugated for target organ delivery. The nanoparticles could be developed fwith one or more of these characteristic based on the requirements. Any such developed nanoparticles could be employed for nanochemoprevention.

Nanomedical approaches to drug delivery centered on developing nanoscale particles or molecules to improve drug bioavailability. [76,77]

Drug delivery focuses on maximizing bioavailability both at specific places in the body and over a period of time. Numerous different strategies have been employed in nanotechnology to optimize drug delivery in a tumor specific manner. This technology extends to different disciplines of science such as chemistry, environmental science and tissue engineering as well as in medicine where it is gradually cementing its position as a potent therapeutic option. Different approaches have been applied to effectively load target drugs to enhance deliveries that are based on the solubility properties of drugs to be loaded. Examples are discussed below.

Nanocurcumin

Curcumin or diferuloylmethane is a yellow polyphenol extracted from the rhizome of turmeric (*Curcuma longa*), a plant grown in tropical Southeast Asia. [78] For centuries, turmeric has been used as a spice and coloring agent for food, as well as a therapeutic agent in traditional medicine. Enthusiasm for curcumin as an anticancer agent has evolved from a wealth of epidemiological evidence suggesting a correlation between dietary turmeric and low incidence of gastrointestinal mucosal cancers. [79] However, like other promising dietary chemopreventive agents, curcumin has not had clinical impact due to its rapid degradation and poor bioavailability in biological systems. [80] Considerable investigations have been performed all around the globe in order to increase curcumin's bioavailability, systemic delivery and its anticancer potential. Numerous nano based attempts have been made and it has been shown that nano loaded curcumin has better bioavailability parameters and efficacy. Earliest attempts on loading the curcumin molecule into nanoparticles came from Plianbangchang et al. where curcuminoids loaded solid lipid nanoparticles (SLNs) were developed using a microemulsion technique at fixed temperatures. [81]

Nanoresveratrol

Resveratrol (3,5,4'-trihydroxy-trans-stilbene) is a phytoalexin produced naturally by several plants when under attack by pathogens such as bacteria or fungi. Resveratrol and its effects are currently a topic of numerous animal and human studies. In mouse and rat experiments, the anticancer, anti-inflammatory, blood sugar lowering and other beneficial cardiovascular effects of resveratrol have been reported. [82] However, most of these results have yet to be replicated in humans. As with other natural chemopreventive agents, resveratrol also has a very short half life and is rapidly glucoronated and sulfonated aiding its rapid turnover and excretion. Therefore, researchers are focused on ways to enhance the bioavailability of resveratrol by different approaches and nano based studies were among the major driving force in this area. The earliest reported nano formulation of resveratrol comes from a study by Yao et al., where they prepared resveratrol chitosan nanoparticles with free amine groups on the surface so as to conjugate ligands, which will actively target special tissues or organs. [83] These chitosan nanoparticles with free amines on the surface were obtained by sodium chloride precipitation through which nanoparticles with different solidification degrees were studied on turbidity, *in vitro* release, encapsulation efficiency, drug loading and diameter. Another liposomal nano based approach was investigated by Wang and group, where they showed that resveratrol release from nanoliposomes *in vitro* fitted the log normal distribution equation and had a property of sustained release. These studies concluded that Res-nanoliposomes could sustain drug release *in vitro* [84].

Epigallocatechin gallate (EGCG) nano formulation

The idea that tea polyphenols, especially the active component EGCG, could have chemopreventive properties came from seminal studies by Mukhtar and group more than a decade ago. [85] Since then, a tremendous research effort has been made in an attempt to decipher the mechanism behind such observed anti-neoplastic effects. Despite promising results in preclinical settings, EGCG clinical applicability to humans has met with limited success, again largely due to inefficient systemic delivery and bioavailability. In the first study of its kind, Mukhtar and group introduced the concept of nanochemoprevention, which uses nanotechnology for enhancing the outcome of chemoprevention. [86]

Genistein nanoencapsulation

Genistein, a soy derived isoflavone, has recently attracted much attention from the medical scientific community. This compound was found to be a potent agent in both prophylaxis and treatment of cancer as well as other chronic diseases. [87,88] The great interest that has been focused on genistein has led to the identification of numerous intracellular targets especially from its action in liver cells. [89] At the molecular level, genistein inhibits the activity of ATP utilizing enzymes such as tyrosine-specific protein kinases, topoisomerase II and enzymes involved in phosphatidylinositol turnover. [90] Moreover, genistein can also act via an estrogen receptor mediated mechanism. [91]

Nano formulations of Taxol (Paclitaxel)

Taxol is among the first clinically and FDA approved chemotherapy drug that originated from natural sources. Its brand name is Paclitaxel. It is a mitotic inhibitor used in cancer chemotherapy. [92] It was discovered from the bark of the Pacific yew tree, *Taxus brevifolia* and thus was named taxol. [93,94] Paclitaxel is water insoluble and is dissolved in Cremophor EL and ethanol as the delivery system. A newer formulation, in which paclitaxel is bound to albumin is sold under the trademark Abraxane. [95]

Summary

Nanotechnology is definitely a medical boon for diagnosis, treatment and prevention of cancer disease. It will radically change the way we diagnose, treat and prevent cancer to help meet the goal of eliminating suffering and death from cancer.

References

[1] Farnebo M, Bykov VJ, Wiman KG. The p53 tumor suppressor: a master regulator of diverse cellular processes and therapeutic target in cancer. Biochemical and Biophysical Research Communications 2010, 396, 85-89.

[2] Linger RJ and Kruk PA. (2010). BRCA1 16 years later: risk-associated BRCA1 mutations and their functional implications. FEBS Letters 2010, 277, 3086-3096.

[3] Weinberg RA. How cancer arises. Scientific American 2006, 275, 62-70.

[4] Pan American Health Organisation, Regional Office of the World Health Organisation (WHO), Cancer (WHO Fact Sheet No. 297), 24/Oct/2006.

[5] Baker Jr JR, Quintana A, Pehlerel L, Banazak-Hollal M, Tomalia D, Raczka E. The synthesis and testing of anticancer therapeutic nanodevices: Biomedical Microdevices 2001, 3(1), 61-69.

[6] Alivisatos P. The use of nanocrystals in biological detection. Nature Biotechnology 2004, 22, 47-52.

[7] Alivisatos AP. Semiconductor clusters, nanocrystals, and quantum dots. Science 1996, 271, 933-937.

[8] Alivisatos AP, Gu WW, Larabell C. Quantum dots as cellular probes: Annual Reviews of Biomedical Engineering 2005, 7, 55-76.

[9] Pinaud F, Michalet X, Bentolila LA, Tsay JM, Doose S, Li JJ, Iyer G, Weiss S. Advances in fluorescence imaging with quantum dot bio-probes. Biomaterials 2006, 27, 1679-1687.

[10] Michalet X, Pinaud FF, Bentolila LA, Tsay JM, Doose S, Li JJ, Sundaresan G, Wu AM, Gambhir SS, Weiss S. Quantum dots for live cells, in vivo imaging, and diagnostics: Science 2005, 307, 538-544 (2005).

[11] Gao XH, Yang LL, Petros JA, Marshal FF, Simons JW, Nie SM. In vivo molecular and cellular imaging with quantum dots: Current Opinion in. Biotechnology 2005, 16, 63-72.

[12] Smith AM, Gao X, Nie S., Quantum dot nanocrystals for in vivo molecular and cellular imaging: Photochemistry and Photobiology 2004, 80, 377-385.

[13] Chan WCW, Maxwell DJ, Gao XH, Bailey RE, Han MY, Nie SM., Luminescent quantum dots for multiplexed biological detection and imaging. Current Opinion in Biotechnology 2002, 13, 40-46.

[14] Harisinghani MG, Barentsz J, Hahn PF, Deserno WM, Tabatabaei S, van de Kaa CH, de la Rosette J, Weissleder R. Noninvasive detection of clinically occult lymph-node metastases in prostate cancer, New England Journal of Medicine 2003, 348, 2491-2499.

[15] Hood JD, Bednarski M, Frausto R, Guccione S, Reisfeld RA, Xiang R, Cheresh DA. Tumor regression by targeted gene delivery to the neovasculature: Science 2002, 296, 2404-2407.

[16] Greider CW and Blackburn EH. Telomeres, telomerase and cancer. Scientific American 1996, 274, 80-85.

[17] Gupta N, Mangal N, Biswas S. Evolution and similarity evaluation of protein structures in contact map space. Proteins: Structure, Function, and Bioinformatics. 2005, 59(2), 196-204.

[18] Rafii-Tabar H and Mansoori GA. Interatomic potential models for nanostructures. Encylopedia of Nanoscience and Nanotechnology 2004, 4, 231-248.

[19] Aquilanti V, Liuti G, Pirani F, Vecchiocattivi F. Orientational and spin—orbital dependence of interatomic forces. Journal of the Chemical Society, Faraday Transactions 2, 1989 85(8), 955-964.

[20] Lebl M and Hachmann J. Peptide synthesis and applications. Methods in Molecular Biology 2001, 298, 167-194.

[21] Davis ME, Chen ZG, Shin DM. Nanoparticle therapeutics: an emerging treatment modality for cancer. National Reviews Drug Discovery. 2008, 7, 771-782.

[22] Petros RA and DeSimone JM. Strategies in the design of nanoparticles for therapeutic applications. National Reviews Drug Discovery 2010 9, 615-627.

[23] Zhang L, Gu FX, Chan JM, Wang AZ, Langer RS, Farokhzad OC. (2008). Nanoparticles in medicine: therapeutic applications and developments. Clinical Pharmacology & Therapeutics 2008, 83, 761-769.

[24] Surh YJ. Cancer chemoprevention with dietary phytochemicals. Nature Reviews cancer 2003, 3, 768-780.

[25] Hampton T. Clinical trials point to complexities of chemoprevention for cancer. Journal of the American Medical Association 2005, 294, 29-31.

[26] Mettlin C. Chemoprevention: will it work? International Journal of Cancer 1997, Suppl 10, 18-21.

[27] Bode AM and Dong Z. Cancer prevention research—then and now. Nature Reviews Cancer 2009, 9, 508-516.

[28] Sporn MB and Newton DL. Chemoprevention of cancer with retinoids. Fed Proc 1979, 38, 2528-2534.

[29] Sporn MB and Liby KT. Cancer chemoprevention: Scientific promise, clinical uncertainty. Nature Clinical Practice Oncology 2005, 2, 518-525.

[30] Liu G, Eggler AL, Dietz BM, Mesecar AD, Bolton JL, Pezzuto JM; van Breemen RB. Screening method for the discovery of potential cancer chemoprevention agents based on mass spectrometric detection of alkylated Keap1. Analytical Chemistry 2005, 77, 6407-6414.

[31] Walsh V and Goodman J. The billion dollar molecule: Taxol in historical and theoretical perspective. Clinical Medicine 2002, 66, 245-267.

[32] Wall ME, Wani MC, Taylor H. Isolation and chemical characterization of antitumor agents from plants. Cancer Treat Rep 1976, 60, 1011-1030.

[33] Wani MC, Ronman PE, Lindley JT, Wall ME. Plant antitumor agents. 18. Synthesis and biological activity of camptothecin analogues. Journal of Medicinal Chemistry 1980, 23, 554-560.

[34] Wani MC, Schaumberg JP, Taylor HL, Thompson JB, Wall ME. Plant antitumor agents, 19. Novel triterpenes from Maprounea africana. Journal of Natural Products 1983, 46, 537-543.

[35]   Wani MC, Nicholas AW, Wall ME. Plant antitumor agents. 23. Synthesis and antileukemic activity of camptothecin analogues. Journal of Medicinal Chemistry 1986, 29, 2358-2363.

[36]   Wani MC, Nicholas AW, Manikumar G, Wall ME. Plant antitumor agents. 25. Total synthesis and antileukemic activity of ring A substituted camptothecin analogues. Structure activity correlations. Journal of Medicinal Chemistry 1987, 30, 1774-1779.

[37]   Xia EQ, Deng GF, Guo YJ, Li HB. Biological activities of polyphenols from grapes. International Journal of Molecular Sciences 2010, 11, 622-646.

[38]   Goswami S.K and Das DK. Resveratrol and chemoprevention. Cancer Letters 2009, 284, 1-6.

[39]   Azmi A.S, Bhat SH, Hadi SM. Resveratrol-Cu(II) induced DNA breakage in human peripheral lymphocytes: Implications for anticancer properties. FEBS Letters 2005, 579, 3131-3135.

[40]   Goel A, Kunnumakkara AB, Aggarwal BB. Curcumin as "Curecumin": From kitchen to clinic. Biochemical Pharmacology 2008, 75, 787-809.

[41]   Surh YJ and Chun KS. Cancer chemopreventive effects of curcumin. Advances in Experimental Medicine and Biology 2007, 595 149-172.

[42]   Banerjee S, Kaseb AO, Wang Z, Kong D, Mohammad M, Padhye S, Sarkar FH, Mohammad RM. Antitumor activity of gemcitabine and oxaliplatin is augmented by hymoquinone in pancreatic cancer. Cancer Research 2009, 69, 5575-5583.

[43]   Banerjee S, Azmi A, Padhye S, Singh MW, Baruah JB, Philip PA, Sarkar FH, Mohammad RM. Structure-activity studies on therapeutic potential of thymoquinone analogs in pancreatic cancer. Pharmaceutical Research 2010, 27, 1146-1158.

[44]   Banerjee S, Padhye S, Azmi A, Wang Z, Philip PA, Kucuk O, Sarkar FH, Mohammad,RM. Review on molecular and therapeutic potential of thymoquinone in cancer. Nutrition and Cancer 2010, 62, 938-946.

[45]   Katiyar SK, Agarwal R, Wang ZY, Bhatia AK, Mukhtar H. (-)-Epigallocatechin-3-gallate in Camellia sinensis leaves from Himalayan region of Sikkim: Inhibitory effects against biochemical

events and tumor initiation in Sencar mouse skin. Nutrition and Cancer 1992, 18, 73-83.

[46] Nihal M, Ahsan H, Siddiqui IA, Mukhtar H, Ahmad N, Wood GS. (-)-Epigallocatechin-3-gallate (EGCG) sensitizes melanoma cells to interferon induced growth inhibition in a mouse model of human melanoma. Cell Cycle 2009, 8 2057-2063.

[47] Ahmad N, Feyes DK, Nieminen AL, Agarwal R, Mukhtar H. Green tea constituent epigallocatechin-3-gallate and induction of apoptosis and cell cycle arrest in human carcinoma cells. Journal of the National Cancer Institute 1997 89, 1881-1886.

[48] Berger SJ, Gupta S, Belfi CA, Gosky DM, Mukhtar H. Green tea constituent (3)-epigallocatechin-3-gallate inhibits topoisomerase I activity in human colon carcinoma cells. Biochemical and Biophysical Research Communications 2001, 288, 101-105.

[49] Singh AK, Seth P, Anthony P, Husain MM, Madhavan S, Mukhtar H, Maheshwari RK. Green tea constituent epigallocatechin-3-gallate inhibits angiogenic differentiation of human endothelial cells. Archives of Biochemistry and Biophysics 2002, 401, 29-37.

[50] Hussain T, Gupta S, Adhami VM, Mukhtar H. Green tea constituent epigallocatechin-3-gallate selectively inhibits COX-2 without affecting COX-1 expression in human prostate carcinoma cells. International Journal of Cancer 2005, 113, 660-669.

[51] Katiyar SK, Afaq F, Perez A, Mukhtar H. Green tea polyphenol (-)-epigallocatechin-3-gallate treatment of human skin inhibits ultraviolet radiation-induced oxidative stress. Carcinogenesis 2001, 22, 287-294.

[52] Boocock D, Patel KR, Faust GE, Normolle DP, Marczylo TH, Crowell JA, Brenner DE, Booth TD, Gescher A, Steward WP. Quantitation of trans-resveratrol and detection of its metabolites in human plasma and urine by high performance liquid chromatography. Journal of Chromatography B Analytical Technologies in the Biomedical and Life Sciences 2007, 848, 182-187.

[53] Anand P, Kunnumakkara AB, Newman RA, Aggarwal BB. Bioavailability of curcumin: Problems and promises. Molecular Pharmacology 2007 4, 807-818.

[54] Freitas Jr RA. What is nanomedicine? Nanomedicine 2005, 1, 2-9.

[55] Freitas Jr RA. Pharmacytes: An ideal vehicle for targeted drug delivery. Journal of nanoscience and Nanotechnology 2006, 6, 2769-2775.

[56] Singh OP and Nehru RM. Nanotechnology and cancer treatment Asian Journal of Experimental Science 2008 22(2), 45-50.

[57] Basu SC and Basu M. (Eds.) (2002) 'Liposome methods and protocols', Methods in Molecular Biology, Humana Press, Totowa, NJ, May.

[58] Silva A, Antonio T, Chung MC, Castro FF, Guido RVC, Ferreira EI. Advances in prodrug design. Mini Reviews in Medicinal Chemistry, 2001, 5(10), 893-914.

[59] Torchilin V and Weissig V. (2003) 'Liposomes: a practical approach', *The Practical Approach Series #264*, Oxford Univ. Press, August 7, Oxford, GB.

[60] Duncan R, Vicent MJ, Greco F Nicholson RI. Polymer-drug conjugates: towards a novel approach for the treatment of endrocine-related cancer. Endocrine-Related Cancer, 2005, 12, S189-S199.

[61] Raj K, Moskowitz B Casciari R. Advances in ferrofluid technology. Journal of Magnetism and Magnetic Materials 1995, 149(1), 174-180.

[62] Lowenstam HA. (1962) 'Magnetite in denticle capping in recent chitons (Polyplacophora). Geological Society of America Bulletin, 1962, 73(4), 435-438.

[63] Lasic DD. Novel applications of liposomes. Trends in Biotechnology 1998, 16, 307-321.

[64] Papahadjopoulos, D, Allen TM, Gabizon A, Mayhew E, Matthay K, Huang SK, Lee KD, Woodle MC, Lasic DD, Redemann C. Sterically stabilized liposomes: Improvements in pharmacokinetics and antitumor therapeutic efficacy. Proceedings of the National Academy of Sciences 1991, 88, 11460-11464.

[65] Winterhalter M and Lasic DD. Liposome stability and formation: Experimental parameters and theories on the size distribution. Chemistry and Physics of Lipids 1993, 64, 35-43.

[66] Lasic DD, Martin FJ, Gabizon A, Huang SK, Papahadjopoulos D. Sterically stabilized liposomes: a hypothesis on the molecular origin of the extended circulation times. Biochimica et Biophysica. Acta 1991, 1070, 187-192.

[67] Hamori CJ, Lasic DD, Vreman HJ, Stevenson DK. Targeting zinc protoporphyrin liposomes to the spleen using reticuloendothelial blockade with blank liposomes. Pediatric Research. 1993, 34, 1-5.

[68] Torchilin VP. Liposomes as targetable drug carriers. Critical Reviews in Therapeutic Drug Carrier Systems. 1985, 2, 65-115.

[69] Elbayoumi TA, Torchilin VP. Liposomes for targeted delivery of antithrombotic drugs. Expert Opinion on Drug Delivery 2008, 5, 1185-1198.

[70] Senior JH. Liposomes *in vivo*: Prospects for liposome-based pharmaceuticals in the 1990s. Biotechnology & Genetic Engineering Reviews 1990, 8, 279-317.

[71] Senior JH. Fate and behavior of liposomes *in vivo*: A review of controlling factors. Critical Reviews in Therapeutic Drug Carrier Systems. 1987, 3, 123-193.

[72] Torchilin VP, Levchenko TS, Lukyanov, AN, Khaw BA, Klibanov AL, Rammohan R, Samokhin GP, Whiteman KR. p-Nitrophenylcarbonyl-PEG-PE-liposomes: Fast and simple attachment of specific ligands, including monoclonal antibodies, to distal ends of PEG chains via p-nitrophenylcarbonyl groups. Biochimica et Biophysica Acta 2001, 1511, 397-411.

[73] Lipinski CA, Lombardo F, Dominy BW, Feeney PJ. Experimental and computational approaches to estimate solubility and permeability in drug discovery and development settings. Advanced Drug Delivery Reviews 2001, 46, 3-26.

[74] Wang J, Mongayt D, Torchilin VP. Polymeric micelles for delivery of poorly soluble drugs: preparation and anticancer activity *in vitro* of paclitaxel incorporated into mixed micelles based on poly(ethylene glycol)-lipid conjugate and positively charged lipids. Journal of Drug Targeting 2005, 13, 73-80.

[75] Siddiqui IA, Adhami VM, Ahmad N, Mukhtar H. Nanochemoprevention: sustained release of bioactive food

components for cancer prevention. Nutrition and Cancer 2010, 62, 883-890.

[76]   Freitas Jr RA. What is nanomedicine? Nanomedicine 2005, 1, 2-9.

[77]   Freitas Jr. Pharmacytes: An ideal vehicle for targeted drug delivery. Journal of Nanoscience and Nanotechnology. 2006, 6, 2769-2775.

[78]   Shishodia S, Sethi G, Aggarwal BB. Curcumin: getting back to the roots. Annals of the New York Academy of Sciences. 2005, 1056, 206-217.

[79]   Aggarwal BB, Kumar A, Bharti AC. Anticancer potential of curcumin: preclinical and clinical studies. Anticancer Research 2003, 23, 363-398.

[80]   Sharma RA, Steward WP, Gescher AJ. Pharmacokinetics and pharmacodynamics of curcumin. Advances in Experimental Medical Biology 2007, 595, 453-470.

[81]   Tiyaboonchai W, Tungpradit W, Plianbangchang P. Formulation and characterization of curcuminoids loaded solid lipid nanoparticles. International Journal of Pharmeceutics 2007, 337, 299-306.

[82]   Jang M and Pezzuto JM. Cancer chemopreventive activity of resveratrol. Drugs Experimental Clinical Research1999, 25, 65-77.

[83]   Yao Q, Hou SX, He WL, Feng JL, Wang XC, Fei HX, Chen ZH. Study on the preparation of resveratrol chitosan nanoparticles with free amino groups on the surface. Zhongguo Zhong Yao Za Zhi (China Journal of Chinese Materia Medica) 2006, 31, 205-208.

[84]   Wang XC, Hou SX, Li W, Li XY, Zhou YW. Study on drug release in vitro and rat intestinal absorption of resveratrol nanoliposomes. Zhongguo Zhong Yao Za Zhi (China Journal of Chinese Materia Medica) 2007, 32, 1084-1088.

[85]   Mukhtar H, Katiyar SK, Agarwal R. Cancer chemoprevention by green tea components. Advances in Experimental Medicine and Biology 1994, 354, 123-134.

[86]   Siddiqui IA, Adhami VM, Bharali DJ, Hafeez BB, Asim M, Khwaja SI, Ahmad N, Cui H, Mousa SA, Mukhtar H. Introducing nanochemoprevention as a novel approach for cancer control: Proof

of principle with green tea polyphenol epigallocatechin-3-gallate. Cancer Research 2009, 69, 1712-1716.

[87] Kumar R, Verma V, Jain A, Jain RK, Maikhuri JP, Gupta G. Synergistic chemoprotective mechanisms of dietary phytoestrogens in a select combination against prostate cancer. Journal of Nutritional Biochemistry 2011, 22(8):723-31

[87] Li W, Frame LT, Hirsch S, Cobos E. Genistein and hematological malignancies. Cancer Letters 2010, 296, 1-8.

[88] Gadgeel SM, Ali S, Philip PA, Wozniak A, Sarkar FH. Genistein enhances the effect of epidermal growth factor receptor tyrosine kinase inhibitors and inhibits nuclear factor kappa B in nonsmall cell lung cancer cell lines. Cancer 2009, 115, 2165-2176.

[89] Szkudelska K, Nogowski L, Szkudelski T. Resveratrol and genistein as adenosine triphosphate-depleting agents in fat cells. Metabolism 2011, 60(5), 720-729.

[90] Yamasaki M, Mukai A, Ohba M, Mine Y, Sakakibara Y, Suiko M, Morishita K, Nishiyama K. Genistein induced apoptotic cell death in adult T-cell leukemia cells through estrogen receptors. Bioscience, Biotechnology and Biochemistry 2010, 74, 2113-2115.

[91] Ganguly, A, Yang H, Cabral F. Paclitaxel-dependent cell lines reveal a novel drug activity. Molecular Cancer Therapeutics 2010, 9, 2914-2923.

[92] Potier P, Gueritte-Voegelein F, Guenard D. Taxoids, a new class of antitumour agents of plant origin: recent results. Nouvelle revue francaise d'hematologie 1994, 36 (Suppl. 1), S21-S23.

[93] Gueritte-Voegelein F, Guenard D, Potier P. Taxol and derivatives: A biogenetic hypothesis. Journal of Natural Products 1987, 50, 9-18.

[94] Miele E, Spinelli GP, Miele E, Tomao F, Tomao S. Albumin-bound formulation of paclitaxel (Abraxane ABI-007) in the treatment of breast cancer. International Journal Nanomedicine 2009, 4, 99-105.

Chemical Carcinogenesis

[1]Dr Nadia Iskandar Zakhary, [2]Dr Abdelfattah Badawi,
[3]Dr Atef T Fahim, [4]Ms Rania Farag Ahmed El-Telbany

[1]Professor of Medical Biochemistry, Cancer Biology Department,
National Cancer Institute, Cairo University, Egypt.
[2]Professor of Applied Organic Chemistry and Medicinal Chemistry,
Petrochemicals Department,
Egyptian Petroleum Research Institute, Cairo, Egypt
[3]Professor of Biochemistry Department,
Faculty of Pharmacy, Cairo University and
Head of Biochemistry Department, October 6 University, Egypt.
[4]Biochemistry Department, Faculty of Pharmacy,
Cairo University, Cairo, Egypt.

Chemical carcinogenesis involves a complex series of events, the earliest of which typically includes DNA damage and the fixation of DNA mutations. Many human cancers are associated with exposure to genotoxic chemicals. There is typically a long period of time (years) between early events that include initial carcinogen exposure, the onset of DNA damage and the fixation of mutations and the subsequent appearance of a tumor. [1]

Diethylnitrosamine

Diethylnitrosamine (DEN) is a representative chemical of a family of carcinogenic N-nitroso-compounds that are known to be activated by liver microsomal p450 enzymes in experimental animals and also in man. DEN has been found in workplaces, processed meats, tobacco smoke and whiskey. [2] It is also derived from metabolism of some therapeutic drugs. It was known to cause perturbations in the nuclear enzymes involved in deoxyribonucleic acid (DNA) repair/replication and is normally used as a carcinogen to induce liver cancer in experimental animal models. [3]

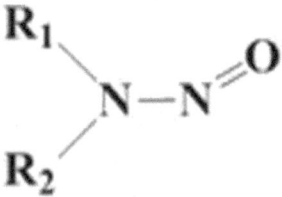

Figure 1. Structure of the nitrosamino group

Diethylnitrosamine has been shown to be metabolized to its active ethyl radical metabolite and the reactive product interacts with DNA causing mutation, which would lead to carcinogenesis. [4]

In liver cancer research using experimental animals, DEN is used either as a complete carcinogen or as an initiator in multistage models. When used as a tumor initiator, DEN is usually given at a single dose of 200 mg/kg to induce pronounced liver necrosis and presumably certain gene mutations in some hepatocytes. [2]

Dialkylnitrosamines after metabolic activation form reactive metabolites that can interact with both oxygen and nitrogen of DNA bases. The formation of reactive oxygen species (ROS) is apparent during the metabolism of DEN resulting in oxidative stress, which may be one of the key factors in the etiology of cancer. [5]

The metabolic pathway of DEN is believed to involve dealkylation by cytochrome p450 2E1 enzymes, followed by the formation of reactive alkyldiazohydroxides and diazonium ions, producing α-hydroxy-N-nitrosopyrrolidine. Subsequent ring opening leads to a cascade of intermediates leading to DNA adducts, thus the p450 is the most important enzyme to be considered in understanding chemical mechanisms of nitrosamine induced carcinogenesis as shown in Figure 2. [6]

Figure 2. The mechanism of DEN toxicity using cytochrome p450. [7]

Carbon tetrachloride

Carbon tetrachloride (CCl_4) is produced industrially by the chlorination of methane, ethane, propene or carbon disulphide. It has been used as a grain fumigant, rodenticide, solvent for oils, fats, rubber cements, resins, fire extinguisher, cleaning agent and has also been used for non-home uses. It was introduced for dry cleaning because of the high cost of the earlier petroleum solvents and this use was discontinued because of its toxicity and corrosiveness. By far its largest usage has been in the manufacture of chlorofluorohydrocarbons (CFH) by reaction with hydrofluoric acid. In turn, these have been used as aerosol propellants, refrigerants and foaming agents but the decreased usage of CFHs and in more recent years, the prohibition of some of these substances has led to very significant reductions in carbon tetrachloride manufacture. [8]

Figure 3. Structure of the carbon tetrachloride.

It has been widely recognized that CCl_4 induced hepatocarcinogenesis is mediated through a cytotoxic proliferative mode of action, since CCl_4 is a potent hepatotoxicant causing generative proliferation of hepatocytes secondary to the cytolethality. [9] The known metabolites of carbon tetrachloride include chloroform, carbon monoxide if oxygen tension is low, carbon dioxide, hexachloroethane and phosgene. The initial step in the liver injury induced by CCl_4 is its cytochrome p450 mediated transfer of a single electron to the C-Cl bond, giving a radical anion as a transient intermediate that eliminates chlorine to form a carbon centered radical. This radical is the trichloromethyl radical ($CCl_3\cdot$) and chloride (Figure 4). The trichloromethyl radical can dismutate to chloroform, bind to macromolecules or attack polyenoic fatty acids in cellular membranes. The double allylic hydrogen atoms in these acids are particularly susceptible to abstraction by free radicals giving chloroform and secondary lipid radicals which react rapidly with molecular oxygen to form lipid peroxyradicals. The trichloromethyl radical can also react with oxygen to form the trichloromethylperoxyl free radical (CCl_3O_2) which is more reactive than the trichloromethyl radical and produces similar kinds of damage. The eventual decomposition of peroxydized fatty acids gives rise to a number of stable end products, such as carbonyls including malondialdehyde, ethane and pentane. [8]

Free radicals induce lipid peroxidation and are believed to be one of the major causes of cell membrane damage leading to a number of pathological situations. In addition, reports on various documented case studies established that CCl_4 produces renal diseases in humans. CCl_4 causes extensive DNA strand breaks and without prompt repair may cause cell death and compensatory cell regeneration. [10]

Figure 4. Metabolic pathways of carbon tetrachloride [8]

Hepatocellularcarcinoma and the immune system

The involvement of the host's immune system in the control of cancer progression has been suspected but remained inconclusive for many years. This is because of the lack of convincing evidence for a direct link between cancer development and lower immune competence in individuals who succumb to cancer. However, standard tests for measuring immune competence to tumor associated antigens, similar to those available for the assessment of responses to bacterial, viral or fungal antigens have not been available. [11]

Innate immunity, which according to the immune surveillance theory, is responsible for early detection and elimination of malignant cells which may be inefficient in patients who develop malignancy. Evidence is convincing that individuals who are older, who have been on immunosuppressive medications over prolonged periods of time or have underlying immune abnormalities, such as an autoimmune disease or a chronic infection (e.g., AIDS) are particularly at risk of malignancy. [11]

Whiteside [11] concluded that members of cancer families have lower levels of natural cytotoxic activity than age matched individuals without cancer in first degree relatives. These studies suggest that among the unaffected family members, persons with lower natural killer (NK) cell activity may be at higher risk of cancer. In combination with evidence for significantly depressed levels of NK cell activity reported for cancer patients with advanced disease, these studies implicate persistently low NK cell activity as a risk for developing malignancy.

Tumors evade the host's immune system

Human tumors, like viruses, have evolved an elaborate assembly of tricks designed to fool the immune system. In fact, molecular mechanisms used by tumors to neutralize immune cells are "borrowed" from viruses. [12] In general, tumors employ two strategies to avoid recognition: they either "hide" from immune cells thus avoiding recognition or they proceed to disable or eliminate immune cells. It has been recognized for a long time that tumors are adept at shedding surface antigens or down regulating expression of key molecules necessary for interactions with immune cells. In this way, tumors can evade the host's immune response by being (a) poor stimulators of T cells or (b) poor targets for tumor-specific T cells. [11]

Interferon gamma

Interferon gamma (IFN-γ), a major effector cytokine of cell immunity, is produced by T-lymphocytes, NK cells or B-lymphocytes and linked to the Janus kinase signal transducer and activator of transcription pathway. IFN is divided into two major subgroups, type-I (α, β, □) and type-II (γ). IFN-γ has various biological effects and previous studies have demonstrated its antiproliferative activity against human cancers. IFN-γ acts specifically on the heterodimeric IFN-γ receptor (IFN-γ R) which has two chains: receptor 1 (IFN-γ R1) and receptor 2 (IFN-γ R2). IFN-γ R1 is expressed on lymphoid cells and various non-lymphoid cells, whereas expression of IFN-γ R2 is high in B-lymphocytes and low or absent in other cell types. [13]

Unlike IFN type-I, type-II (IFN-γ) possesses very marked pleiotropic immunomodulating, rather than antiviral activity. In fact, in many immunoregulating activities namely antiviral protection, cell growth regulation and modulation produce induction of class I major histocompatability complex (MHC) antigens. IFN-γ is active at lower concentrations than other interferons. Type-II (IFN-γ) has been reported to augment monocyte tumoricidal activity, hydrogen peroxide generation, monocyte antibody-dependent cellular cytotoxicity and both class I and class II MHC. [14] Its role in the expression of immunologically diverse molecules including a constant fraction of immunoglobulins and complement factor receptors is of great significance. It is capable of enhancing the expression and action of different soluble inflammatory mediators, such as tumor necrosis factor alpha (TNF-α), interleukin I (IL-I) and IFN-γ. [15]

Malaguarnera [15] have emphasized the cytokines' central role in defending the host against viral infections whereas new reports support the marked involvement of cell immunity during evolution towards chronic HCV. These considerations imply that similar to what occurs in HBV infection, determination of IFN-γ concentrations may be useful in evaluating the host's immunological response. Since the marked antigenic polymorphism characteristic of HCV and other factors linked to the host's immunological reaction appears to be responsible for the evolution of chronic HCV, the IFN-γ regulated immune response to evaluate its role in the prognosis and evolution of the disease.

Interferon gamma is a key molecule involved in deviation of T-helper cells to the T helper cell 1 (Th1) pathway and down regulation of IFN-γ R2 contributes to counteracting the biological effects resulting from Th1 deviation. It was shown that IFN-γ induces self-resistance by down regulating IFN-γ R2 in the situation of murine helper T-cell differentiation. There have been very few reports about the expression of IFN-γ receptors in HCC cells. If IFN-γ receptors are expressed on the surface of hepatocelluar carcinoma cells and the expression of IFN-γ receptors can be enhanced by certain stimuli, then the anti-proliferative effect of IFN-γ could be a promising new chemotherapeutic approach for HCC. [13]

Reversal of immune dysfunction and cancer immunotherapy

Traditionally, cell mediated biotherapies used in treating cancer patients have been aimed at increasing these responses via activation, amplification of proliferation or re-population of the host with *ex vivo* activated antitumor effector cells. These strategies referred to as active or passive cellular immunotherapy respectively have undergone considerable refinement over the years. Active as well as passive immunotherapy of cancer have the best opportunity to succeed in the setting of minimal residual disease, with attenuation of apoptosis of activated tumor specific T cells and establishment of long lived antitumor memory responses. Also, restoration of normal lymphocyte homeostasis is probably an important component of such immunotherapy. In addition, cytokines play a key role in regulation of lymphocyte survival. [11]

Hepatocellular carcinoma and oxidative stress

The relationship between cancer and oxidative stress has been the subject of intensive debate. This has been mainly due to the well documented fact that the cancer cells are under high levels of oxidative stress compared to normal cells. In the past decades oxidative stress has been linked both in the etiology and the potential treatment of cancer. [16] Vitaglione et al. [17] reported that as the oxidative stress plays a central role in liver disease pathogenesis and progression. The use of antioxidants as therapeutic agents as well as drug coadjuvants has been proposed to counteract liver damage. Reactive oxygen species (ROS), reactive nitrogen species (RNS) and free radicals are constantly formed in the human body and removed by an antioxidant defense system. A certain amount of ROS/ RNS production is in fact necessary for proper health. For example ROS/ RNS help the immune system to eliminate microorganisms. In healthy individuals, the generation of ROS/RNS appears to be approximately in balance with antioxidant defense. An imbalance between ROS/RNS and antioxidant defenses in favor of the former via excessive production of ROS/NOS, loss of antioxidant defenses or both have been described as oxidative/nitrosative stress. [18]

There are both endogenous and exogenous sources of ROS generation as shown in Figure 5. Endogenous sources include those resulting from (i) mitochondrial oxidative phosphorylation, (ii) p450 metabolism, (iii) peroxisomes and (iv) activation of inflammatory cells. It has been postulated that during oxidative phosphorylation 1-2% of molecular oxygen is converted to ROS primarily through a series of sequential one, two and three electron reductions giving rise to superoxide, hydrogen peroxide and hydroxyl radical formation consecutively. [19] In addition, activation of p450 metabolism has been proposed as a very significant source of ROS formation by mechanisms that involve (i) redox cycling, (ii) peroxidase catalyzed drug oxidations and (iii) "futile cycling" of cytochrome p450. In particular, induction of p450 2E1 and 2B has been proposed to contribute significantly to ROS formation primarily through metabolism of ethanol and phenobarbital respectively. Furthermore, in a number of studies using chemicals such as peroxisomes proliferators, an increased production of hydrogen peroxide was observed that contributed to increased levels of oxidative stress and their association with cancer induction. Finally, inflammatory cells like neutrophils and macrophages are perhaps the most significant sources of endogenous ROS formation. More specifically, activated macrophages through "respiratory burst" give rise to various ROS and primarily superoxide and hydrogen peroxide. For instance, activation of specialized macrophages in the liver known as Kupffer cells has been implicated in tumor promotion through ROS release. [20] On the other hand, exogenous sources of ROS generation include those of various xenobiotics with a variable degree of potency, chlorinated compounds, various transition metals participating in Fenton-type chemical reactions and radiation. All of which have been documented to cause ROS-induced damage to cellular macromolecules namely DNA, RNA, lipids and proteins, both in vitro and in vivo. [21]

Figure 5. Reactive oxygen species production and disruption of cellular homeostasis.

ROS can be produced by both endogenous and exogenous sources. An overload of the normal antioxidant defense system by these reactive oxygen molecules will result in oxidative stress and eventual oxidative damage to critical cellular macromolecules. Abbreviations: CAT, catalase; GSH, reduced glutathione; GSHperox, reduced glutathione peroxidase; SOD, superoxide dismutase; VitC, vitamin C; VitE, vitamin E. [22]

Consequence of oxidative stress

The elevated oxidative stress in cells can lead to the modification of number of cellular targets and cause cell damage and death. The most important of these targets include (i) nuclear and mitochon-drial DNA, single strand breaks, (ii) damage of mitochondrial inner membrane, which can lead to loss of cellular stores of ATP and (iii) damage of membrane phospholipids, with the initiation of lipid peroxidation. [23]

Lipids are most susceptible macromolecules and are present in the plasma membrane in the form of polyunsaturated fatty acids (PUFA). The ROS attack PUFA in the cell membrane leading to a chain of chemical reactions called lipid peroxidation. The various pathways of lipid peroxidation are shown in this Figure 6. The reaction occurs in three distinct steps: (i) initiation, (ii) propagation and (iii) termination. During initiation, the free radicals react with the fatty acid chain and release lipid free radicals. This lipid radical further reacts with molecular oxygen to form lipid peroxyl radicals. Peroxyl radicals again react with fatty acid to produce lipid free radicals and this reaction is propagated. During termination, the two radicals react with each other and the process comes to an end. This process of fatty acid breakdown produces hydrocarbon gases namely ethane and pentane as well as aldehydes. [23]

Figure 6. Various pathways of lipid peroxidation.

The methylene groups of polyunsaturated fatty acids are highly susceptible to oxidation and their hydrogen atoms. After the interaction with the radical, R• are removed to form carbon-centred radicals 1• - reaction 1. Carbon centred radicals react with molecular dioxygen to form peroxyl radicals - reactions 2 and 3. If the peroxyl radical is located at one of the ends of the double bond - 3• - , it is reduced to a hydroperoxide which is relatively stable in the absence of metals - reaction 4. A peroxyl radical located in the internal position of the fatty acid, 2•, can react by cyclisation to produce a cyclic peroxide adjacent to a carbon centred radical - reaction 5. This can then either be reduced to form a hydroperoxide - reaction 6 - or through reaction 7 it can undergo a second cyclisation to form a bicyclic peroxide which after coupling to dioxygen and reduction yields a molecule structurally analogous to the endoperoxide. Compound 7 is an intermediate product for the production of malondialdehyde - reaction 8. Malondialdehyde can react with DNA bases G, A, and C to form adducts M1G, MA and M1C - reactions 9-11. Peroxyl radicals located in the internal position of the fatty acid - 2•1 - can, besides cyclisation reactions, - reaction 5 - also abstract hydrogen from the neighbouring fatty acid molecule, creating thus lipid hydroperoxides - reaction 12. They can further react with redox metals (e.g. iron) to produce reactive alkoxyl radicals - RO•, reaction 13 - which, after cleavage - reaction 14 - may form, e.g. gaseous pentane; a good marker of lipid peroxidation. [24]

Cancer and oxidative stress

Sources of ROS in preneoplasias and tumors

It has been estimated that nearly 20% of the global human cancers are attributable to infective and inflammatory diseases. [25] The most important cancers with infection etiology are gastric cancer due to *Helicobacter pylori gastritis*, hepatocelluar carcinoma due to chronic HBV or HCV infection of the liver or bladder cancer due to liver infestation by *Schistosoma haematobium*. [26] The activated inflammatory cells in these conditions induce oxidant generating enzymes, e.g. NADPH oxidase, myeloperoxidase and inducible nitric oxide synthase. This mechanism is responsible for the production of high concentrations of different ROS. Furthermore, it must be kept in mind that the most important sources of ROS are the electron transport chains of mitochondria and endoplasmic reticulum. [26]

Cells in preneoplastic stages and cancer cells are metabolically active and need high levels of ATP supply to maintain their high proliferation rates which compared to normal tissue, are increased. The high energy production in the mitochondrial respiration chains is associated with increased ROS production. This is the second important source of ROS in cancer tissue. [27]

Involvement of oxidative stress in carcinogenesis

In general, the multistage process of carcinogenesis involves the distinct phases of initiation, promotion and progression. The cellular and molecular events underlying each of these phases include DNA damage, increased proliferation, deficient cell death and further genetic instability, respectively as shown in Figure 7. [28]

Figure 7. Multistage process of cancer and role of ROS. [27]

However, there are a number of studies indicating that oxidative DNA damage alone could not account entirely for tumor development. It has been shown that elevated levels of 8-hydroxyguanine do not reflect increased cancer rates. [29] The question arises then, what other mechanisms could account for the involvement of ROS in carcinogenesis? ROS can affect a number of cellular processes critical in tumor development, such as cell proliferation, senescence, inflammation and metastasis. In terms of cell proliferation, ROS have been shown to modulate cell cycle regulation through modulation of various cell cycle proteins including p53. [30] ROS have also been shown to modulate the cell death (senescence) process [31] by acting either as an anti-senescence stimulus [32] or through the specific induction of apoptosis-inducing factor (AIF) which induces apoptosis and consequently maintains the transformed phenotype of a cancer cell. [33] On the other hand, inflammation has long been known to act as a trigger in cancer development. For example, chronic hepatitis B viral infection and elevated liver levels of 8-OHdG can lead to development of hepatocellular carcinoma. [34]

Finally, metastasis is an integral part of tumor progression during which ROS have been documented to play a major role [13] In fact, various studies have shown that metastatic tumor cells produce higher levels of ROS than primary malignant cells which together with increasing levels of ROS metabolizing enzymes and antioxidant compounds greatly reduce metastasis. [35]

In conclusion

Diethylnitrosamine and carbon tetrachloride are the most prominant chemical carcinogens causing mutation which lead to hepatocellular carcinoma due to reactive oxygen species production, disruption of cellular homeostasis and consequence oxidative stress

References

[1]   Poirier CM. Chemical-induced DNA damage and human cancer risk. Nature Reviews Cancer 2004. 4: 630-637.

[2]   Liao JD, Blanck A, Eneroth P, Gustafsson J, Hallstrom PI. Diethylnitrosamine causes pituitary damage, disturbs hormone levels and reduces sexual dimorphism of certain liver functions in the rat. Environmental Health Perspectives 2001, 109(9), 943-947.

[3]   Sierra ML, Tosal L, Nivard JM, Comendadora A, Vogel W. The importance of distinct metabolites of N-nitrosodiethylamine for its in vivo mutagenic specificity. Mutation Research—Reviews 2001, 483, 95-104.

[4]   Sheweita AS and Mostafa HM. Nitrosamines and their effects on the level of glutathione, glutathione reductase and glutathione S-transferase activitiesin the liver of male mice. Journal of Cancer Letters 1996, 99, 29-34.

[5]   Wills PJ, Suresh V, Arun M, Asha VV. Antiangiogenic effect of Lygodium flexuosum against N-nitrosodiethylamine-induced hepatotoxicity in rats. Chemico-Biological Interactions 2006, 164(1-2), 25-38.

[6]   Yamazaki H, Yukiharu I, Yun CH, Guengerich FP, Shimada T. Cytochrome P450 2E1 and 2E6 enzymes as major catalysts for metabolic activation of N-itrosodialkylamines and tobacco-related nitrosamines in human liver microsomes. Journal of Carcinogenesis 1992, 13, 1789-1794

[7]   Novak I and Kovac B. (2007): Nitrosamines: A challenge for theory and experiment. Chemical Physical Letters 2007, 445, 129-132.

[8]   McGregor D and Lang M. (1996): Carbon tetrachloride: genetic effects and other modes of action. Journal of Mutatation Research 1996, 366(3), 181-95.

[9]   Tsujimura K, Ichinose F, Hara T, Yamasaki K, Otsuka M, Fukushima S. The inhalation exposure of carbon tetrachloride promote rat liver carcinogenesis in a medium-term liver bioassay. Toxicology Letters 2008, 176(3), 207-214.

[10]   Khan MR, Rizvi W, Khan GN, Khan RA, Shaheen S. Carbon tetrachloride-induced nephrotoxicity in rats: protective role of Digera muricata. J Ethnopharmacol. 2009, 122(1), 91-99.

[11]   Whiteside tl. Immune suppression in cancer: Effects on immune cells, mechanisms and future therapeutic intervention. Seminars in Cancer Biology 2006, 16(1), 3-15.

[12]   Lybarger L, Wang X, Harris M, Hansen TH. Viral immune evasion molecules attack the ER peptide-loading complex and exploit ER-associated degradation pathways, Current Opinion in Immunology 2005, 17, 71-78.

[13]   Okada S, Ishikawa N, Shirao K, Kawaguchi H, Tsumura M, Ohno Y, Yasunaga S, Ohtsubo M, Takihara Y, Kobayashi M. The novel IFNGR1 mutation 774del4 produces a truncated form of interferon-gamma receptor 1 and has a dominant-negative effect on interferon-gamma signal transduction. Journal of Medical Genetics, 2007, 44(8), 485-491.

[14]   Schroder K, Hertzog JP, Ravasi T, Hume AD. Interferon gamma an overview of signals, mechanisms and functions. Journal of Leukocyte Biology 2004, 75, 163-189.

[15]   Malaguarnera M, Di Fazio I, Laurino A, Pistone G, Restuccia S, Trovto BA Decrease of interferon gamma serum levels in patients with chronic hepatitis C. Biomedical & Pharmacology Journal 1997, 51(9), 391-396.

[16]   Pervaiz S and Clement MV. Tumor intracellular redox status and drug resistance-serendipity or a causal relationship. Journal of Current Pharmaceutical Design 2004, 10, 1969-1977.

[17]   Vitaglione P, Morisco F, Caporaso N, Fogliano V. Dietary antioxidant compounds and liver health. Critical Reviews in Food Science and Nutrition 2004, 44(7-8), 575-586.

[18]   Dalle-Donne I, Rossi R, Colombo R, Giustarini D, Milzani A. Biomarkers of oxidative damage in human disease. Journal of Clinical Chemistry 2006, 52, 601-623.

[19]   Pappa A, Franco R, Schoneveld O, Galanis A, Sandaltzopoulos R, Panayiotidis MI. Sulfur-containing compounds in protecting against oxidant-mediated lung diseases. Current Medicinal Chemistry 2007, 14(24), 2590-6.

[20]   Klaunig JE, Kamendulis LM. The role of oxidative stress in carcinogenesis. Annual Reviews of Pharmacology and Toxicology 2004, 44, 239-267. del Río LA, Sandalio LM, Corpas FJ, Palma JM, Barroso JB. Reactive oxygen species and reactive nitrogen species in peroxisomes. Production, scavenging and role in cell signaling. Plant Physiology 2006, 141(2), 330-335.

[21]   Klaunig JE, Xu Y, Isenberg JS, Bachowski S, Kolaja KL, Jiang J, Stevenson DE, Walborg Jr EF. The role of oxidative stress in chemical carcinogenesis. Environmental Health Perspectives 1998, 106(Suppl 1), 289-295.

[22]   Agarwal A Prabakaran AS. Mechanism of measurement and prevention of oxidative stress in male reproductive physiology. Indian Journal of Experimental Biology, 2005, 43, 963-974.

[23]   Valko M, Rhodes CJ, Moncol J, Izakovic M, Mazur M. Free radicals, metals and antioxidants in oxidative stress-induced cancer. Chemico-Biological Interactions 2006, 160, 1-40.

[24]   Parkin DE, Warraich Q, Fleming DJ, Chew GK, Cruickshank ME. An audit of the quality of endometrial cancer care in a specialized unit. Scottish Medical Journal 2006, 51(2), 22-24.

[25]   Roessner A, Kuester D, Malfertheiner P, Schneider-Stock R. Oxidative stress in ulcerative colitis-associated carcinogenesis. Journal of Pathology—Research and Practice; 2009, 204, 511-524.

[26]   Pelicano H, Carney D, Huang P. ROS stress in cancer cells and therapeutic implications. Drug Resistance Update 2004, 7(2), 97-110.

[27]   Halliwell B. Oxidative stress and cancer: have we moved forward. Biochemical Journal 2007, 401, 1-11.

[28]   Arai T, Kelly VP, Minowa O, Noda T, Nishimura S. The study using wild-type and Ogg1 knockout mice exposed to potassium bromate shows no tumor induction despite an extensive accumulation of 8-hydroxyguanine in kidney DNA, Journal of Toxicology, 2006, 221, 179-186.

[29]   Bensaad K, Vousden KH. Savior and Slayer: the two faces of p53. Nature Medicine 2005, 11, 1278-1279.

[30]   Chandra J, Samali A, Orrenius S. Triggering and modulation of apoptosis by oxidative stress. Free Radical Biology and Medicine 2000, 29, 323-333.

[31]   Vaquero EC, Edderkaoui M, Pandol SJ, Gukovsky I, Gukovskaya AS. Reactive oxygen species produced by NAD(P)H oxidase inhibit apoptosis in pancreatic cancer cells. Journal of Biological Chemistry 2004, 279, 34643-34654.

[32]   Urbano A, Lakshmanan U, Choo PH, Kwan JC, Ng PY, Guo K, Dhakshinamoorthy S, Porter A. AIF suppresses chemical stress-induced apoptosis and maintains the transformed state of tumor cells. EMBO Journal 2005, 24, 2815-2826.

[33]   Hagen TM, Huang S, Curnutte J, Fowler P, Martinez V, Wehr CM, Ames BN, Chisari FV. Extensive oxidative DNA damage in hepatocytes of transgenic mice with chronic active hepatitis destined to develop hepatocellular carcinoma. Proceedings of the National Academy of Sciences of the USA 1994, 91, 12808-12812.

[34]   Heirman I, Ginneberge D, Brigellius-Flohe R, Hendricks N, Agostinis P, Brouckaert P, Rottiers P, Grooten J. Blocking tumor cell eicasonoid synthesis by GPx4 impedes tumor growth and malignancy. Free Radical Biololgy and Medicine 2006, 40, 285-294.

The Role of Some Natural and Synthetic Compounds in Cancer Protection

[1]Dr Nadia Iskandar Zakhary, [2]DrAbdelfattah Badawi,
[3]DrAtef T Fahim, [4]Ms Rania Farag Ahmed El-Telbany

[1]Professor of Medical Biochemistry, Cancer Biology Department,
National Cancer Institute, Cairo University, Egypt.
[2]Professor of Applied Organic Chemistry and Medicinal Chemistry,
Petrochemicals Department,
Egyptian Petroleum Research Institute, Cairo, Egypt
[3]Professor of Biochemistry Department,
Faculty of Pharmacy, Cairo University and Head of Biochemistry
Department, October 6 University, Egypt.
[4]Biochemistry Department, Faculty of Pharmacy,
Cairo University, Cairo, Egypt.

1-α-lipoic acid

Lipoic acid (LA) is a widely occurring coenzyme found in prokaryotic and eukaryotic microorganisms as well as in animals and plants. [1] Lipoic acid (1,2-dithiolane-3-pentanoic acid, 1,2-dithiolane-3-valeric acid or thioctic acid) is a sulfur containing coenzyme and in its reduced form the dihydrolipoic acid (DHLA, 6,8-dimercaptooctanoic acid or 6,8-thioctic acid) contains two thiol groups per molecule. (Figure 1)

Figure 1. Chemical structures of lipoic and dihydrolipoic acids.

Lipoic acid plays a pivotal role in energy metabolism. It is involved in different multienzyme complexes such as pyruvate dehydrogenase, α-ketoglutarate dehydrogenase and glycine decarboxylase complex. [2] It is reduced to DHLA, which is subsequently reoxidised by lipoamide dehydrogenase with the formation of NADH. Overall, LA and DHLA act as a redox couple, carrying electrons from the substrate of the dehydrogenase to NAD. [3]

The antioxidant potential of LA and DHLA has been highlighted. Usually antioxidant substances possess antioxidant properties in their reduced form. LA is unique among antioxidant molecules because it retains protective functions in both its reduced and oxidized forms [4] although DHLA is the more effective one in performing antioxidant functions. In addition, the relatively low molecular mass of LA (206 daltons), larger than ascorbic acid but much smaller than tocopherol makes it soluble in both water and fat so that it is a molecule which connects the activity of antioxidants in the membranes with that of antioxidants in the cytoplasm strengthening the antioxidant network of the cells. [3]

Another reason for its dual solubility resides in the chemical structure of the molecule (Figure 1). The carboxylic acid end group renders it more water soluble than tocopherol. At the same time, LA and DHLA have more carbon atoms than ascorbic acid and this makes them more soluble in lipophylic membrane compartments. [3] Hence, LA is of interest because it is known to scavenge hydroxyl radicals, singlet oxygen, hydrogen peroxide, hypochlorous acid, peroxynitrite and nitric oxide. DHLA also quenches peroxyl and superoxide radicals making the ALA/DHLA redox couple one of the most powerful biological antioxidant systems. [5] **(Wollin and Jones, 2003).**

Antioxidant activity is a relative concept. It depends on the kind of oxidative stress and the oxidative substrate. According to Packer *et al.* [4] upon evaluating the antioxidant potential of a compound, criteria such as

- specificity of the free radical scavenging
- interaction with other antioxidants
- metal chelating activity
- effects on gene expression
- bioavailability
- location (in aqueous or membrane domains or both)
- ability to repair oxidative damage have to be taken into consideration.

Due to its redox potential, DHLA can reduce GSSG to GSH and cystine to cysteine (CSSC to CSH) but GSH and CSH cannot reduce LA to DHLA. Cysteine is transported to the cells more efficiently than cystine and is promptly used as sources for GSH synthesis. LA has been found to be a moderate antioxidant and DHLA, a good antioxidant in particular and the ability of DHLA to inhibit LPO has been reported. [3]

An antioxidant needs only to meet a few of the previous mentioned criteria to play an important role in the detoxification of oxidative stress. An 'ideal' antioxidant would fulfil all the above criteria. The LA /DHLA redox couple approaches the ideality. It can be considered the 'universal antioxidant'. The two thiol groups present in DHLA provide this unique reactivity pattern. [3]

Selenium

Selenium (Se) is a metalloid trace element with atomic number 34 and melting point of about 220.5 °C and boiling point at about 684.9 °C. It belongs to the sulfur family of elements, which also includes oxygen, tellurium and polonium and has some common properties with sulfur, including valency. [6]

Selenium is physiologically essential in small amounts but can be toxic in larger amounts. It is known today that humans and animals require Se for the normal function of a number of Se dependent compounds. Se levels in the body are mainly dependent on the amount of selenium in the diet. It is present in both vegetable and animal products. The amount of selenium in food is a function of the selenium content of the soil. Se enters the food chain while incorporated into plant proteins as the amino acids L-selenocysteine and L-selenomethionine, as well as some inorganic forms of selenium. [7] There are several seleno compounds in the tissues of plants, animals and seafood. Different Se concentrations can be found in foods from different geographical areas, mainly due to variations in the total Se content in soil even in the same country as well as its variable availability to plants. There is a wide variation in the Se content in plants. The main reason is that plants do not appear to require Se. Seleno compounds found in food areas as follows [7]

- selenate which is the major inorganic compound found in both animal and plant tissues
- selenocysteine which is the predominant seleno amino acid in tissues when inorganic selenium is given to animals
- selenomethionine which is the major seleno compound found initially in animals given this selenoamino acid and is converted with time to selenocysteine
- selenium methylselenocysteine which is the major seleno compound in selenium enriched plants such as garlic, onions, broccoli florets and sprouts and wild leeks as shown in Figure (2).

Figure 2. Proposed pathways for the metabolism of biologically important selenomolecules.

CH_3SeH is methylselenol, $(CH_3)_2SE$ is dimethylselenide, $(CH_3)_3SE^+$ is trimethylselenonium, H_2Se is hydrogen selenide, SeO_2 is selenium dioxide, SeP is selenoprotein P, SeW is selenoprotein W and tRNA is transfer RNA. [8]

Biological Functions of Selenoproteins

Selenium is an integral part of more than about 30 known proteins. These proteins are called selenium containing proteins or selenoproteins, of which approximately 15 have been purified to allow characterization of their biological functions. [9]

Selenium is found in human and animal tissues as L-selenomethionine or L-selenocysteine. Only a small fraction of L-methionine in proteins is present as L-selenomethionine. On the other hand, the incorporation of L-cysteine into selenoproteins is not random. Namely, in contrast to L-selenomethionine, which randomly substitutes for L-methionine, L-selenocysteine does not randomly substitute for L-cysteine. [10] Selenoproteins perform a variety of physiological roles. Selenoproteins are composed as follows [7]

- four selenium-dependent glutathione peroxidases (GSHPx1, GSHPx2, GSHPx3 and GSHPx4)
- three selenium-dependent iodothyronine deiodinases
- three thioredoxin reductases (selenium is at the active site of the enzyme)
- selenoprotein P
- selenoprotein W
- selenophosphate synthetase.

Another class of selenoproteins are the iodothyronine deiodinase enzymes (type 1, 2, and 3 iodothyronine deiodinases) which catalyze the 5'-mono deiodination of the prohormone thyroxin (T4) to the active thyroid hormone 3,3',5-triiodothyronine (T3), thus regulating the thyroid hormone metabolism. All three different selenium dependent iodothyronine deiodinases can both activate and inactivate thyroid hormone, making selenium an essential element for normal development, growth, and metabolism through regulation of thyroid hormones. [11]

Thioredoxin reductase is a recently identified selenocysteine containing enzyme which catalyzes the NADPH dependent reduction of thioredoxin and therefore plays a regulatory role in its metabolic activity.

Among other things, the thioredoxin reductases reduce intramolecular disulfide bonds and participate in the regeneration of several antioxidant systems including vitamin C. Maintenance of thioredoxin in a reduced form by thioredoxin reductase is important for regulation of cell growth and viability. [12]

Selenoprotein P is an extracellular protein that contains 10 selenium atoms per molecule as selenocysteine and may serve as a transport protein for selenium. Approximately 60% of selenium in plasma is incorporated in selenoprotein P. The function of selenoprotein P has not been clearly delineated. Since it is also expressed in other tissues, it has been suggested to function as a transport protein, as well as an antioxidant capable of protecting endothelial cells from damage by a RNS called peroxynitrite. It associates with endothelial cells, probably through its heparin binding properties. [13]

Selenoprotein W is found in muscles and it is thought to play a role in muscle metabolism. [14] Selenophosphate synthetase catalyzes the synthesis of monoselenium phosphate, a precursor of selenocysteine which is required for the synthesis of selenoproteins. Incorporation of selenocysteine into selenoproteins is directed by the genetic code and requires the enzyme selenophosphate synthetase. [7]

Epidemiological studies, preclinical investigations and clinical intervention trials support the role of selenocompounds as potent cancer chemopreventive agents [15] especially for several major cancers, including prostate, lung, colon and liver cancers. [16] Accumulated evidence has suggested that the dose and the chemical structure are important determinants of chemopreventive activities of Se compounds. [17] Recent attention has been focused on intracellular-signaling cascades as common molecular targets for cancer chemoprevention.

Cysteine

Cysteine (Cys) is an α-amino acid with the chemical formula $NH_2\text{-}CH(CH_2SH)\text{-}CO_2H$. It is a nonessential amino acid which means that humans can synthesize it. With a thiol side chain, Cys is classified as a hydrophilic amino acid. Because of the high reactivity of this thiol, Cys is an important structural and functional component of many proteins and enzymes. In animals, biosynthesis begins with the amino acid serine. The sulfur is derived from methionine, which is converted to homocysteine through the intermediate S-adenosylmethionine. Cystathionine beta synthase then combines homocysteine and serine to form the asymmetrical thioether cystathionine. The enzyme cystathionine gamma lyase converts the cystathionine into Cys and alpha ketobutyrate as shown in Figure 3. [19] Although classified as a non-essential amino acid, in rare cases Cys may be essential for infants, the elderly and individuals with certain metabolic disease or who suffer from malabsorption syndromes. Cysteine can usually be synthesized by the human body under normal physiological conditions if a sufficient quantity of methionine is available. It is potentially toxic and is catabolized in the gastrointestinal tract and blood plasma. In contrast, cystine travels safely through the GI tract and blood plasma and is promptly reduced to the two cysteine molecules upon cell entry. Cysteine is found in most high protein foods including animal sources such as pork, sausage meat, chicken, turkey, duck, luncheon meat, eggs, milk, whey protein, ricotta, cottage cheese and yogurt. Vegan sources include red peppers, garlic, onions, broccoli, brussels sprouts, oats, granola and wheat germ. [19]

Figure 3. Known biosynthetic pathways to cysteine.

The transulfuration pathway in animals: three reactions [20] involving methyl transfer:

- conversion of S-adenosylmethionine (SAM) to homocysteine
- condensation of homocysteine with serine to cystathione
- cystathione is cleavaged to cysteine

N-acetyl-L-cysteine (NAC) is a derivative of Cys where an acetyl group is attached to the nitrogen atom. This compound is sometimes considered as a dietary supplement, although it is not an ideal source since it is catabolized in the gut. NAC is often used in cough medicines because it breaks up the disulfide bonds in the mucus and thus liquefies it making it easier to cough up. NAC is also used as a specific antidote in cases of acetaminophen overdose. [21]

Due to the ability of thiols to undergo redox reactions, Cys has antioxidant properties. Cysteine antioxidant properties are typically expressed in the tripeptide glutathione which occurs in humans as well as other organisms. The systemic availability of oral glutathione (GSH) is negligible, so it must be biosynthesized from its constituent amino acids—cys, glycine and glutamic acid. Glutamic acid and glycine are readily available in most western diets but the availability of Cys can be the limiting substrate. [22]

The sulfide in iron sulfur clusters and in nitrogen compounds is extracted from cysteine which is converted to alanine in the process. [21] Beyond the iron sulfur proteins, many other metal cofactors in enzymes are bound to the thiolate substituent of cysteinyl residues. Examples include zinc in zinc fingers and alcohol dehydrogenase, copper in the blue copper proteins, iron in cytochrome P450, and nickel in the [NiFe]-hydrogenases. The thiol group also has a high affinity for heavy metals so that proteins containing cysteine will bind metals such as mercury, lead, and cadmium tightly. [23]

The most important property of Cys is that it is readily capable of acting as an antioxidant with respect to the reactive oxygen species such as superoxide, peroxyradicals and hydroxyl radicals. The mechanism of this interaction involves the formation of the cystine dimer via the thyl radicals. The dimer can be reduced back to the cysteine through an appropriate 2 electron reduction such that cysteine can continue to moderate radical toxicity. Cysteine can also mop up harmful oxidants such as HOCl and HOBr. The efficiency of cysteine as a radical and oxyhalogen scavenger is related to the rate at which it reacts with radicals, oxyhalogens and halogens. Thus, Cys should be preferentially oxidized over cell tissue for it to act as an antioxidant. [19]

Germanium

Germanium (Ge) as an element was identified in 1886 as a semi metal. It exists in some plants and it is used in Chinese medicine to treat some diseases and found in health promoted foods. As the organic germanium electronic structure and configuration enable it to carry out many tasks it has a healing effect on the body, including the neutralization and elimination of toxic substances, removal of free radical and protection of blood cell from radiation. [24]

For most people the major source of germanium uptake is through food. It is present in practically all foods, although only at very low levels. Many of the earlier reported values of the concentrations of Ge in some medicinal plants such as ginseng, aloe or garlic are in the high ppm range. [25] Some Ge containing organic compounds such as car-boxyethylgermanium sesquioxide have attracted considerable attention because of their potential for numerous clinical applications as anticancer drugs. Organic Ge and coordinative Ge compounds display analgesic, hypotensive, fungistatic, bactericidal, antiviral, antimalarial and radio protective effects. [26]

In both humans and animals Ge has been shown to increase INF-□ in the blood, activate macrophages and natural killer cells, bring blood hemoglobin levels up and white cell counts down, stimulate immunomodulation activity in the B cell system and demonstrate antitumor and antiviral activities. Ge therefore, may be an excellent adjuvant immunochemotherapeutic agent. The effects of Ge on various immune parameters are almost identical to that of known INF-□ immunomodulating activity [27] In addition, studies on immune suppressed animals and on patients with malignancies or rheumatoid arthritis suggest that Ge normalized the function of T cells, B lymphocytes, antibody dependent cellular cytotoxicity, natural killer cell activity and numbers of antibody forming cells. Obviously Ge has a "normalizing" influence on the immune system. Our bodies have many physical/chemical systems that are in a state of "homeostasis", which is the ability to restore systems to their "normal" state. A substance that assists the body systems to restore to normality is called an "adaptogen". Thus Ge is without any question described as an adaptogen. [27]

Conclusion

Recent attention has been focussed on the significant cancer chemopreventive activities of α-lipoic acid, selenium, cysteine and germanium compounds.

References

[1] Busby RW, Schelvis JPM, Yu DS, Babcock GT, Marletta MA: Lipoic acid biosynthesis: LipA is an iron-sulfur protein. Journal of the American Chemical Society 1999, 121, 4706-4707.

[2] Gueguen V, Macherel D, Jaquinod M, Douce R, Bourgui-gnon J. Fatty acid and lipoic acid biosynthesis in higher plant mitochondria. Journal of Biological Chemistry 2000, 276, 5016-5025.

[3] Navari-Izzo F, Quartacci MF, Sgherri C. Lipoic acid: a unique antioxidant in the detoxificationof activated oxygen species. Journal of Plant Physioliology and Biochemistry 2002, 40, 463-470.

[4] Packer L, Witt EH, Tritschler HJ. Lipoic acid as biological antioxidant. Journal of Free Radical Biology and Medicine 1995, 19, 227-250.

[5] Wollin DS and Jones HJP. (2003): Lipoic acid and Cardiovascular Disease. Journal of Nutrition 2003, 133, 3327-3330.

[6] Rayman MP (2000): The importance of selenium to human health. The Lancet. 2000, 15, 356(9225), 233-41.

[7] Dodig S and Cepelak I. The facts and controversies about selenium. Acta Pharmaceutica 2004, 54, 261-276.

[8] Zeng H and Combs Jr GF Jr. Selenium as an anticancer nutrient: roles in cell proliferation and tumor cell invasion. Journal of Nutritional Biochemistry 2008, 19(1), 1-7.

[9] Jameson RR and Diamond AM. A regulatory role for Sec tRNASerSec in selenoprotein synthesis. RNA 2004, 10(7), 1142-1152.

[10] Brown KM and Arthur JR. (2001): Selenium, selenoproteins and human health: a review. Public Health Nutrition 2001, 4, 593-599.

[11]   Larsen PR, Davies TF, Hay ID. (1998): The Thyroid Gland in Williams Textbook of Endocrinology. 9th ed. (Eds. J. D. Wilson, D. W. Foster, H. M. Kronenberg and P. R. Larsen), W. B. Saunders Company, Philadelphia, pp. 389-515.

[12]   Mustacich D and Powis G. Thioredoxin reductase, 2000 J. Biochemistry 2000, 346, 1-8.

[13]   Burk RF, Hill KE, Motley AK. (2003): Selenoprotein metabolism and function: evidence for more than one function for selenoprotein Nutrition 2003, 133, 1517S-1520S.

[14]   Whanger PD (2000): Selenoprotein W: A review, Cell Journal of Molecular Life Sciences 2000, 57, 1846-1852.

[15]   El-Bayoumy K and Sinha R. (2004): Mechanisms of mammary cancer chemoprevention by organoselenium compounds. Journal of Mutation Research 2004, 551, 181-97.

[16]   Yu SY, Zhu YJ, Li WG. (1997): Protective role of selenium against hepatitis B virus and primary liver cancer in Qidong. Biological Trace Element Research 1997, 56, 117-124.

[17]   Abdulah R, Miyazaki K, Nakazawa M, Koyama H. (2005): Chemical forms of selenium for cancer prevention. Journal of Trace Elements in Medicine and Biololoy 2005, 19, 141-150.

[18]   ChenT and Wong Y. Selenocystine induces reactive oxygen species mediated apoptosis in human cancer cells. Journal Biomedicine & Pharmacotherapy 2009 Biomedicine & Pharmacotherapy 2009, 63:105-113.

[19]   Darkwa J, Mundoma C, Simoyi HR. (1998): Antioxidant chemistry Reactivity and oxidation of DL-cysteine by some common oxidants. Journal of the Chemical Society, Faraday Transactions 1998, 94(14), 1971-1978.

[20]   Kitabatake M, So MW, Tumbula DL, Söll D. (2000): Cysteine biosynthesis pathway in the archaeon Methanosarcina barkeri encoded by acquired bacterial genes. Journal of Bacteriology 2000, 182(1), 143-145.

[21]   Lill R and Mühlenhoff U. (2006): Iron-sulfur protein biogenesis in eukaryotes: components and mechanisms. Annual Review of Cell and Developmental Biology, 2006, 22, 457-86.

[22]   Murray RK, Granner DK, Rodwell VW. (2000): in Harper's Biochemistry. Twenty-fourth edition, Appleton & Lange Publisher. p. 221& 648.

[23]   Baker DH and Czarnecki-Maulden GL. (1987): Pharmacologic role of cysteine in ameliorating or exacerbating mineral toxicities. Journal of Nutrition 1987, 117(6), 1003-1010.

[24]   Hassan EF, El-Sayef JM, Hafiz AA. (2001): Organic germanium a new additive to gutta-percha root canal filling material. Cairo Dental Journal, 2001, 17, 201-204.

[25]   Omae, I. (1999):in Applications of Organometallic Compounds, J. Wiley & Sons, Chichester, 165-184.

[26]   Choudhary MA, Mazhar M, Ali S, Song, X, Eng G. Synthesis and characterization of diphenyltin (IV) dicarboxylates containing germanium. Journal of the Chinese Chemical Society 2005, 52: 463-470.

[27]   Levine AS. Organic germanium a novel dramatic immunostimulant. Journal of Orthomolecular Medicine. 1987, 2(2), 83-87

Germanium Against Cancer

[1]Dr Eman Noaman and [2]Dr Abdelfattah Badawi

[1]Professor Laboratory of Biochemistry Radiation Biology,
International Center for Radiation Research and Technology
Nasr City, PO Box 29, Cairo, Egypt.
[2]Professor, Laboratory of Surfactants, Egyptian Petroleum
Research Institute, Heliopolis, PO Box 5051,
Cairo 11771, Egypt.

Introduction

Organic germanium compounds are recognized as nutritional supplements. Germanium is rapidly becoming a significant trace mineral because of its safety and versatile range of therapeutic properties which have enabled it to achieve "miraculous" remissions and cures, particularly in the hands of the Japanese, who have had the most experience with this element. [1-4]

The effects of germanium are sometimes remarkable for this semi-metal which comes out of the earth and is present everywhere. Organic germanium's electronic structure and configuration enable it to carry out many tasks which have a healing effect on the body. [4] These effects include the elimination and neutralization of toxic substances such as CCl_4 [5] and free radicals. [4] Germanium also protects blood cells from radiation. [6] At the molecular level it has unambiguously documented that organic germanium has immune enhancing properties. [4,7] This was confirmed in a study on the antiviral activity of germanium (IV) sodium ascorbate (GeNaA) that was investigated by the author Badawi. [8] This germanium compound was submitted to U.S. Army Medical Research Insititute of Infectious Diseases, Fort Detrick, Frederick, Maryland, USA. The study was concerned with a reverse transcriptase (RT) assay for the human immunodeficiency virus (HIV). GeNaA was found to significantly inhibit RT in vitro suggesting AIDS retarding activity. [8] Organic germanium's immune enhancing properties were also noted in a number of studies particularly in the case of cancer and arthritis. [2,6,9]

Organic germanium has been used in a broad spectrum of regimes, both on its own with diet and stress counseling and as a drug in cancer trials in conjunction with chemotherapy, radiation therapy and surgery. [10,11]

There are normally several distinct stages whereby a potential cancer drug is tested before it can be made available. If the substance demonstrates anticancer activity in a number of *in vitro* assays, then studies on animals will follow. If these studies demonstrate promising results, then experiments and trials will be conducted with human cancer patients. Organic germanium could be found as a natural substance with virtually no demonstrated toxicity.

Germanium is classified as a food supplement and not a drug, which has enabled faster progress in establishing its therapeutic action in humans for many diseases including cancer. Thus, treatment of human cancer patients with germanium has occurred in parallel with the careful scientific studies in animals, establishing its anticancer action which resulted in a wealth of documentation from both human side, as well as laboratory data, [4]

Cancer research studies on three organogermanium compounds namely Ge-132, Sanugerman and spirogermanium, at the cellular level in animals and human cancer patients, have produced positive evidence for the potential of organogermanium compounds having anticancer properties.

Cellular level

The in vitro cytotoxic activity and other biological effects of Spirogermanium which represent chemical class of compounds exhibiting antitumor activity that has been studied *in vitro*. Increasing drug concentrations and longer exposure times were shown to have an exponential greater killing effect on NIL 8 hamster cells. Cytotoxicity was temperature dependent. "Quiescent" cultures were significantly less sensitive to Spirogermanium than with logarithmically growing cells. These lethal effects showed no phase specificity. There was no evidence of progression delay through the cycle following Spirogermanium treatment. When Spirogermanium was tested against a range of human cell lines, the consistency of the values for the drug concentration required to reduce survival by 50% on the exponential part of the survival curve was most marked. The survival curves, characterized by an initial shoulder, were steep and exponential with measurements over a narrow concentration range. This was carried out as a complete cell lysis occurred at levels causing a greater than 2-log kill. Cell membrane damage by Spirogermanium, as judged by dye exclusion. Damage was progressive with time and increasing drug concentrations. Protein synthesis proved most susceptible to the drug. Spirogermanium concentrations cytotoxic to tumor cells. Such concentrations were also toxic to cultured rat neurons, confirming the clinical neurological toxicity encountered. The precise mode of action of Spirogermanium remains to be established and these data further illustrate its apparent lack of specify. [12]

Tests with various laboratory cancerous cell lines demonstrated that Spirogermanium is not a phase or cell cycle specific drug. It inhibits DNA, RNA and protein synthesis with protein synthesis being the most susceptible to this agent. Spirogermanium has shown cytotoxic activity *in vitro* against several human tumor cell lines and cultured rat neurons. Although Spirogermanium has no effect on normal bone marrow colony forming cells in mice, dogs or man, it has revealed cytotoxic activity *in vitro* against human myeloid leukemia cell line K 562 at clinically achievable concentrations. These *in vitro* findings indicate selective cytotoxic activity against leukemic cells, suggesting that this drug is a candidate for clinical studies in acute and chronic leukemias. [13-14]

A series of analogs of Spirogermanium (germanium containing azaspirane) were synthesized and evaluated in a number of *in vitro* studies to define the structure-activity relationships of this class of compounds relative to their potential therapeutic activities. In a colony-forming assay using HT-29 human colon carcinoma cells, various analogs in which carbon replaced germanium retained the potent cytotoxic activity *in vitro* was seen with spirogermanium. Increased cytotoxic potency within the group of carbon containing analogs was directly related to the increase in the length of the alkyl group(s) attached to the carbon atom opposite to the azaspirane ring structure. DNA and protein synthesis by HT-29 cells were inhibited by these compounds. However, inhibition occurred only at supralethal concentrations or after long exposure times with the drug. The effect of these compounds on macrophage cell function was evaluated *in vitro* by their ability to modulate superoxide (O_2^-) production by macrophages. Spirogermanium inhibited the production of O_2^- by activated macrophages in the HT-29 colony formation assay. The results demonstrate that with this class of compounds, *in vitro* cytotoxic activity does not appear to be a direct result of the inhibition of macromolecular synthesis and that macrophage function can be modulated *in vitro* at non-cytotoxic concentrations. [15]

The oncostatic activity of potential anticancer substances were measured by the allium test, using activity dividing plant cells. Sanumgerman when analyzed by this procedure showed the characteristics of an active oncostatic compound. [16,17] Some studies on the organic germanium's mode of action at the cellular and molecular level showed that germanium compounds inhibited viral (HSV-l) replication *in vitro* and blocked the synthesis of DNA in hepatoma 22A and ovarian cancer cells. [12,18]

The anticarcinogenic effects of bioginseng and two germanium selective drugs produced by cultivating cells of Ginseng radix (Panax ginseng C. A. Mey) in media containing organogermanium compounds revealed an inhibitory effect on the development of squamous cell carcinomas of the uterus cervix and vagina which were induced chemically by intravaginal applications of 7,12-dimethyl benz-(a)-anthracene in mice. [19]

Antiproliferative properties have been detected for the non-platinum group metal antitumor agents. These are represented by non-platinum group metal antitumor agents that are represented by inorganic and organometallic compounds containing either the main group metals such as gallium, germanium and tin or transition metals such as titanium, vanadium, iron, copper and gold. In the case of germanium complexes, the antitumor activity is obviously not based on direct cytotoxic effects but on host mediated immune potentiating mechanisms. [20]

Animal studies

Antitumor activity of sanumgerman studies with several types of cancer revealed good results. In the group of mice receiving Sanumgerman, the incidence of tumor was decreased from 50% in control to 20% in treated group. [20] Also Sanumgerman increased the survival rates when administered to mice with colon carcinoma. [21] In other studies, Sanumgerman showed prophylactic effect against colon, lung and myeloma type cancer. [22]

Spirogermanium is azaspirane, an antitumor agent with the metal germanium substituted for a one carbon moiety in the ring structure. This drug has curative *in vivo* antitumor activity against ascetic Walker 256 carcinosarcoma in rats. No hematologic toxicity was recorded during the preclinical toxicologic evaluation. [23]

(Ge-132) has shown significant antitumor activity against a wide spectrum of tumors which has been shown to be mediated by inactivation of immune mechanism, including macrophage, natural killer cells (NK), interferon (INF) and T suppressor cells. In a murine model, it has been shown that the antitumor activity of Ge-132 can be depleted by administration of macrophage (M phi) blockers. [24] Oral administration of Ge-132 in mice was demonstrated to be effective in activating M phi (Ge-132-cytotoxic M phi). The cytotoxic activity of the M phi macrophages appeared in the peritoneal cavity of mice 48 hours after the oral administration of the compound. On cultivation of RL male-1 leukemia or Ehrlich carcinoma cells with Ge-132-cytotoxic, macrophage fractions obtained from PEC of Ge-132-treated mice exhibited an inhibitory effect against certain tumors both *in vitro* and *in vivo* suggesting that the antitumor effect of Ge-132 observed *in vitro* resulted from the activation of M phi. [24] In another study, mice treated orally with Ge-132 exhibited antitumor activity against Ehrlich (allergenic) and RL 1 (synergenic) ascites tumors in BALB/c mice. Sera obtained from mice 24 hours after Ge-132 administration displayed the highest antitumor effect and the antitumor activity was dose-dependent. Sera prepared from mice 12, 36 or 48 hours after Ge-132 treatment had no protective effect. Circulating interferon (IFN) was induced at 24 hours after administration. These results suggest that the antitumor activity in the sera of Ge-132-treated mice may have been expressed through IFN-gamma. [25] The antitumor effect of (Ge-132) was also examined in mice using two systems: one was the ascetic form of Ehrlich carcinoma in DDI mice and the other was the solid form of Meth-A fibrosrcoma in BALB/c mice. In the mice with Ehrlich ascetic tumors, a remarkable prolongation in life span was observed. The cytotoxic macrophages (Mo) were induced in the peritoneal cavity after intraperitoneal (i.p.) or oral (p.o.) administration of Ge-132 (300 mg/kg) but not after intravenous (i.v.) injection of the same compound. When the *in vivo* effect of these *in vitro* active of Mo was examined after adoptive transfer to mice bearing Ehrlich ascetic tumor cells, a significant antitumor effect was noted. In the mice bearing solid Meth-A tumors, i.v. injections of Ge-132 (100 mg/kg) were found to inhibit tumor growth remarkably. This inhibitory effect of Ge-132 by i.v. administration was explained by the continued augmentation of NK activity in peripheral blood, which was followed by the induction of specific killer cells appearing in the spleen. When the mice which had recovered from Meth-A tumor growth, following i.v. injections of Ge-132 were challenged with the same tumor; all mice were able to tolerate the challenge but not a challenge of RL male 1 tumor cells. These observations may indicate that the varied antitumor effects of Ge132 when different administration methods were used, can be explained by the variation in effectors cells induced by such different administration routes. [26] The antitumor effect of combining immunochemotherapy with Ge-132 and an antitumor agent was studied using C57BL/6 mice bearing Lewis lung carcinoma (3LL) on 3LL local tumor growth. Pulmonary metastases, survival, delayed type hypersensitivity (DTH) and body weight in tumor bearing mice were obtained. Inhibition of tumor growth in the combined groups enhanced antimetastatic effect, prolonged survival time and recovery of loss of both DTH end body weight. Adoptive transfer of Ge-132 stimulated spleenocytes in 5-fluorourcil (5-FU) treated mice bearing 3LL also obtained these antitumor effects. These results therefore suggest that the effects of Ge-132 were expressed through modification of immunocytes. Furthermore, Ge-132 enhanced the antitumor activity of bleomycin as well as that of 5-FU. These facts suggested that Ge-132 is useful for antitumor combination immunochemotherapy. [27]

The administration of IFN-containing sera (IFN-sera) obtained from Ge-132-treated mice (Ge-mice) or the passive transfer of macrophages (M phi) to mice bearing ascites tumors, resulted in the inhibition of tumor growth. The cooperative role of IFN-sera and Ge-M phi in the display of Ge-132-antitumor activity was studied. When mice were pretreated with antimouse IFN gamma antiserum, no IFN-inducing or antitumor activities of the compound were detected. Cytotoxic activities were detected in peritoneal M phi of mice treated with Ge-sera and passive transfer of M phi to tumor-bearing mice resulted in the inhibition of tumor growth. When tumor-bearing mice were pretreated with substances toxic to M phi, no antitumor activity of Ge-sera was observed. However, Ge-132 antiturnor activity was observed in mice depleted of T-cells even though the antitumor effects of the compound itself were not demonstrable in T-cell-depleted mice. Therefore, a part of the antitumor activity of Ge-132 appears to be expressed as follows: Ge-132 stimulates T-cells to produce circulating lymphokine(s) which were inactivated by anti-IFN gamma treatment. Activated M phi were generated from resting M phi by these lymphokine(s). The transplanted tumors are inhibited by the M phi. [28]

Non platinum group metal antitumor agents represented by inorganic and organometallic compounds were investigated for their antitumor activity. Their antiproliferative properties have been detected. The spectrum of antitumor activity was not identical with that of cytostatic platinum complexes. In case of germanium complexes, the antitumor activity is obviously not based on direct cytotoxic effects but rather on host mediated immunopotentiating mechanisms. [20] In the same manner, the antitumor activity of the following four metallocene compounds were tested against Ehrlich ascites tumor in female CF1 mice: decaphenylstannocene ['η^5-$(C_6H_5)_5C_5$]2Sn(II(, decabenzylstannocene ['η^5-$(C_6H_5CH_2)_5C_5$]2Sn(II(, decaphenylgermanocene [the main group IV elements tin or germanium as the central metal atom] [['η^5-$(C_6H_5)_5C_5$]$_2$Ge(II) and decabenzylgermanocene ['η^5-$(C_6H_5CH_2)_5C_5$]2Ge(II(. These compounds all contained two penta substituted cyclopentadienyl ring ligands in a sandwich arrangement. The complexes caused cure rates of 40% to 90% of the animals treated over rather broad dose ranges. With both of the germanocene complexes, no strong dose activity relationship was manifested. The toxicity of all four metallocenes was low. The LD10 values of both stannocenes was 460 and 500 mg/kg and those of both germanocenes were higher than 700 mg/kg. Regarding the isolated pentasubstituted cyclopentadiene ligands $(C_6H_5)_5C_5H$ and $(C_6H_5CH_2)_5C_5H$, they also exhibited antitumor activity which was less pronounced than that of the metal containing sandwich complexes. Decasubstituted stannocene and germanocene compounds represent a non platinum group of metal antitumor agents that are structurally different from the well known inorganic and organometallic cytostatics. [29]

The pulmonary metastasis of Lewis lung carcinoma was strongly blocked by daily intraperitoneal (i.p.) treatment with novel organic compound (PCAGeS) for 7 days after tumor implantation. The metastasis preventive activity of PCAGeS was markedly reduced when mice were treated with carrageenan as a macrophage blocker. On the other hand, treatment with antiasialo GM1 antiserum did not significantly affect the percentage of inhibition of metastasis by the compound. These results suggest that macrophages rather than natural killer NK cells play an important role in the suppression of metastasis by PCAGeS. Oral administration PCAGeS induced tumoristatic end tumoricidal activities in the peritoneal macrophages of mice. The activity of NK cells was also augmented by i.p. treatment with this compound. These results suggest that PCAGeS is a useful substance for preventing pulmonary metastasis. [30]

Research on the effect of different kinds of germanium compounds on 1,2-dimethylhydrazine induced intestinal cancer in rats, revealed that natural organic germanium has the best preventive effect for intestinal cancer (P < 0.01), followed by organic germanium (P < 0.05). Inorganic germanium had no effect. However, there is no difference in the cancer prevention effect of germanium when provided one month before and during dimethylhydrazine treatment and during dimethylhydrazine treatment only. [31]

The modifying potential of carboxyethylgermanium sesquioxide (GE), allyl sulfide (AS) and indole-3-carbinol (I3C) on lesion development was examined in a wide-spectrum initiation model. AS treatment significantly decreased the incidence of hepatic hyperplastic nodules, adenoma of the lung and thyroid as well as papillary or nodular hyperplasia of the urinary bladder. Administration of GE also significantly inhibited the development of hepatic nodules and adenoma of the lung and thyroid. However, I3C only inhibited the hyperplastic nodules of the liver. These results demonstrated that this multi organ initiation model could be useful in confirming the organ specific modification potential and in addition, the inhibitory effect of AS, I3C and GE on liver, lung, thyroid and urinary bladder carcinogenesis. [32]

Investigation on the effect of Ge-132 on the generation of splenic suppressor macrophages (S-M phi) in C3H/He mice (H-2k) immunized with allogeneic spleen from C57Bl/6 mice (H-2b) indicated that Ge-132 could regulate cytotoxic T lymphocyte (CTL) generation in all immunized mice by preventing the generation of I-J antigen expression on macrophages (I-J+S-M phi). [33] The administration of a combination of Ge-132 and lipolysaccharide (LPS) on Meth-A sarcoma bearing mice was attempted. In addition to the induction of tumor necrosis factor in sera (TNF) as a multidisciplinary cancer therapy (TNF therapy) per se, the potential on the above parameters by employing immunothermotherapy was coupled with regional hyperthermia treatment. This immunothermotherapy enhanced the antitumor effects produced by the above TNF therapy. [34]

The effect of Ge-132 as an interferon-gamma (IFN-gamma) inducer on post surgical immunosuppression was evaluated from the immunological response augmented in canine neutrophils, macrophages and peripheral blood lymphocytes (PBL) using the chemiluminescence technique. It appeared that the generated free radical, which blocked the phagocytosis of macrophages and PBL was activated by IFN-gamma. The results suggest that Ge-132 pre-treatment may be efficacious and useful in preventing the multifaceted clinical symptoms induced by postoperative immunosuppression in dogs. [35]

The anticarcinogenic effects of bioginseng and two germanium selective drugs produced by cultivating cells of ginseng radix (Panax ginseng, C. A. Mey) in a conventional medium or in media containing organogermanium compounds were studied. Squamous cell carcinomas of the uterus cervix and vagina were induced by intravaginal applications of 7,12-dimethylbenz-(a)-anthracene in mice. The drugs of ginseng were used orally or intravaginally during a long period of time of the post initiation stage of carcinogenesis. All the drugs used locally inhibited effectively the development of induced carcinomas of the uterus, cervix and vagina. When used orally, the ginseng drugs exhibited only an insignificant tendency to inhibit the carcinogenesis of uterus, cervix and vagina. The anticarcinogenic effects of the compared drugs were similar. [36]

Protective effects of spirulina Ge-132 and vitamin E on colon aberrant crypts induced by 1,2-dimethylhydrazine (DMH) were observed. Results showed Spirulina powder, Ge-132 and vitamin E all could inhibit the function of aberrant crypts of colon. In the ninth week during multiple injection with DMH, a lot of aberrant crypts of colon had been induced and a certain amount of aberrant crypts foci had been generated. The number of aberrant crypts and aberrant crypts foci was significantly less in animals protected by spirulina than in positive controls (P < 0.01) but there was no significant difference between them during 21st and 24th week of injections. [37]

Yeast selenium (YSe) and Ge-132 were administered respectively in the drinking water of Wister rats after and during the administration of N-methyl-N'-nitrosoguanidine (MNNG) administered also in their drinking water to induce the precancerous lesion in stomach. The results showed that the incidence of glandular stomach cancer in the YSe group was significantly lower than that in the control group. The infiltrating depth of glandular stomach cancer in the YSe group and the Ge-132 group was remarkably shallower than that in the control group. These findings suggest that Yse and Ge-132 have some preventive effect on the precancerous lesion in rat glandular stomach induced by MNNG. [38]

Propagermanium (3-oxygermylpropionic acid polymer) is an organic germanium compound that activates the immune system. The action of propagermanium on T-cell-mediated murine hepatic injury induced by concanavalin A (Con A) has been investigated. Oral administration of propagermanium inhibited the development of liver injury about 10 h after Con A injection. Histological analysis demonstrated that propagermanium attenuated the extent of liver damage compared with controls, reducing infiltration by leucocytes, especially CDllb-positive cells. Infiltration by CD4-positive cells was not affected. Tumor necrosis factor (TNF)-alpha and interferon (IFN)-gamma are crucial for the development of hepatitis in this model. Propagermanium treatment induced significant inhibition of subsequent TNF-alpha production about 10 h after Con A injection without affecting IFN-gamma, interleukin (IL)-10, IL-4 and IL-12 production. This effect on TNF-production coincided with the inhibition of aminotransferase activity late in the progression of Con A-induced liver injury. These facts suggest that propagermanium affects the macrophage (Mphi) function in the liver sinusoid. These results might explain the mechanisms by which propagermanium inhibits Con-A-induced liver injury; that is, propagermanium improves hepatitis through mechanisms including the reduced production of TNF-alpha, without modification of Thl- and Th2-cell function. [39]

Propagermanium compound has immunopotentiating activity. One study showed the hepatoprotective effect of propagermanium and its mechanism in an experimental animal model of acute liver injury induced with Corynebacterium parvum (C. parvum) and lipopolysaccharide (LPS) injection. Oral pretreatment with propagermanium decreased alanine aminotransferase (ALT) and aspartate aminotransferase (AST) activity in a dose dependent manner. Significant attenuation of ALT and AST activity was obtained at a dose of 3 mg/kg. Administration of propagermanium also inhibited the infiltration of mononuclear cells into the liver of mice induced by C. parvam/LPS. In this animal model, blood cytokine levels increased rapidly after LPS injection causing severe hepatitis. It is noteworthy that tumour necrosis factor-alpha (TNF-alpha) and interferon-gamma (IFN-gamma) are important mediators of the progress of liver injury. Propagermanium reduced IFN-gamma production by 53% at a dose of 3 mg/kg and also significantly inhibited the production of interleukin-12 (IL-12). These results indicate that propagermanium inhibits cell infiltration in the liver and cytokine production and improves massive liver injury in C. parvurn/LPS mice. [40]

Clinical trials

Clinical trials and use in private practice for more than a decade have demonstrated germanium's efficacy in treating a wide range of serious afflictions including cancer. [41]

Clinical trials on lung cancer have shown a statistically significant effect of Ge-132 on life prolongation and tumor regression as well as overall improvement in performance status and immunological parameter. [42] A double blind controlled for unresectable lung cancer was commenced in 1980. The patients were divided into classes depending on the type of cancer. The treatment consisted of either chemotherapy or a placebo or administer double blind. This meant that neither the patients nor the doctor knew whether the individual was receiving germanium or placebo. Final results have revealed a significant difference between the placebo and germanium in the proportion of partial and complete patient responses to the treatment with organic germanium. [42]

A phase 1 clinical trail was conducted with 35 patients with a variety of cancers with intravenously administered Spirogermanium. This trial was conducted in order to define a tolerated dosage and to determine the anticancer activity. Several of the patients experienced mild transient side effects such as dizziness which was all resolved within a few minutes to several hours. There was neither evidence of cumulative toxicity nor of bone marrow depression. One patient showed a partial response in the palpable nodes for two months. [23]

In phase II trial, 18 heavily pretreated patients with advanced ovarian malignancy were treated with Spirogermanium, 11 i.m. and 7 i.v. Objective responses (partial remission) were obtained in two (11%) of the 18 patients with a remission duration of 5 and 23 months respectively. An additional four (22%) patients had stable disease. Each of these six patients had a better quality of life and there were few side effects. Myelosuppression, nausea or other gastrointestinal side effects did not occur. The investigation showed that Spirogermanium is useful as a palliative chemotherapeutic agent in patients with advanced ovarian malignancy. [43]

A report in the clinical studies mentioned that Spirogermanium is remarkable for its lack of bone marrow toxicity as confirmed by preclinical toxicology and clinical studies. Moderate, predictable and reversible CNS toxicity were dose limiting. Activity against malignant lymphoma, ovarian cancer, breast cancer, large bowel cancer and prostatic cancer was reported in this clinical study. The drug has been under clinical investigation against the wide spectrum of solid tumors and malignant lymphomas. [44]

A phase II study of Spirogermanium was conducted in a series of 15 patients with metastatic prostatic carcinoma. All the patients have previously received multiple hormonal therapies. The drug was administered at the dose of 200 mg/m^2 by continuous infusion for five days, and 120 mg/m^2 and then three times a week subsequently. The side effects were mainly neurological toxicity and phlebitis at the injection points which were dose and schedule dependent. Only one partial response for two months was noted in this series. Thus, Spirogermanium seems to have a limited value in patients with prostatic cancer. [45]

Seventeen patients with advanced colorectal carcinoma were treated with a combination of 5-fluorouracil and Spirogermanium (azaspirane-germanium compound) which is remarkable for its lack of hematologic, gastrointestinal, renal or hepatic toxicity. Response to treatment as well as the incidence and severity of toxicity were evaluated. No patient achieved a complete response and there were only three partial responses. Toxicity was unexpectedly frequent and severe. One patient was removed from study early due to intractable diarrhea and there were two toxic deaths, both attributable to neutropenia and sepsis. Significant toxicity occurred in all seventeen patients, including three instances of Grade 3 or 4 hematologic toxicity. Given the low response rate and high incidence of life threatening toxicity, it was not recommended that further evaluation be carried out for this schedule of 5-fluorouracil and Spirogermanium in the treatment of colorectal carcinoma. [46]

Spindle cell carcinoma (SCC) is a rare form of lung cancer representing 0.2 to 0.3% of all primary pulmonary malignancies. Even with combined surgery, chemotherapy, and radiation therapy these tumors are associated with a poor prognosis and only 10% of patients survive 2 years after diagnosis. A woman patient was described an unresectable SCC who did not respond to conventional treatment with combined modality therapy. She chose to medicate herself with daily doses of germanium obtained from a health food store. The patient prompted symptomatic improvement and remained clinically and radiographically free of disease for 42 months after starting her alternative therapy. [47]

These few case histories represent a small fraction of the 'anecdotal' evidence that has accumulated attesting to organic germanium's therapeutic effectiveness in treating cancer. Not all cancer patients receiving organic germanium have been cured. Minimal therapeutic effects have been noted in several clinical trials with intravenously administered Spirogermanium. This may in part reflect the trial selection and administration procedures. However, almost invariably a general overall improvement in the quality of occurs due to organic germanium's ability to relieve pain.

Recent investigations

Novel amino acid germanates were investigated as immunumodulators. [48,49] The selected amino acids used were histidine, methionine and glutathione. It was found that both bis-methionino germanate and bis-glutathiono germanate significantly increased the levels of serum IL-12 and IFN-6 by mechanisms which act as neuro chemical messengers to the immuno system that might provide sufficient immune response to cancer diseases in future research.

Novel cationic germanium metal based surfactants were recently investigated for their cytotoxic activities. [50] The obtained data revealed that the isothiouronium tin based germanium surfactactant displayed low toxicity in human normal lymphocytes and high cytotoxicity in human cell lines leukemia lymphoblastic NALM-6 cells, promyelogtic HL-60 cells and breast adeno carcinoma MCF-7 cells.

Conclusion

Germanium is present in all living plant and animal matter in micro trace quantities. Its therapeutic attributes include immuno-enhancement, oxygen enrichment, free radical scavenging and analgesia and heavy metal detoxification. Toxicological studies documented germanium's rapid absorption and elimination from the body, and its safety.

We could conclude from the previous findings that the future use of new germanium compounds to treat neoplastic diseases without adverse effects has some exciting possibilities.

References

[1]   Aso H, Suzuki F, Yamaguchi T, Hayashi Y, Ebina T, Ishida N. Induction of interferon and activation of NK cells and macrophages in mice by oral administration of G-132, an organic germanium compound. Microbiology and Immunolology 1985, 29, 65-74.

[2]   Suzuki F, Brutkiewicz RR, Pollard RB. Importance of T-cell and macrophages in the antitumor activity of carboxyethyl germanium sesqui oxide (G-132). Anticancer Research 1985, 5, 479-83.

[3]   Takoshima R and Mitsui Y. Germanium as a stabilizer of cysteine eye drops. In: Immunomodulation by Microbiology. Products and related synthesis compounds. In: Sym. Osaka Yamamura and Kotani (eds) 1981, 27-29.

[4]   Asai K. Miracle Cure. Organic Germanium, Japan Publications Inc, 1980.

[5]   Zakhary NI, Abdel-Hamid NA, El-Aaeser AA, Badawi A, Sharawi, S, Kamal Sh. The role of germanium citrate lactate in the protection of liver injury, Metal Ions in Biology & Medicine (III), John Libbey, Eurotext. 1994, 343-357.

[6]   Abu-Ghader AR, Osman SA, Badawi AM, Hassan AB. Effect of Sanumgerman on antioxidant system of whole body gamma irradiated mice. In CB Medical Treatment Sym. (II), Spiez, Switzerland, 1996, 40-42.

[7]   Mizushima Y, Shoji Y, Kaneko K. Restoration of impaired immunoresponse by germanium in mice. International Archives of Allergy and Immunology 1980, 63, 338-339.

[8]   Badawi AM. Inhibitory effect of germanium (IV) sodium ascorbate on the in-vitro reverse transcriptase of human immunnodeficiency virus. In: Metal Ions in Biology and Medicine. Collery Ph, Poirier

LA, Manfait M, Etienne JC, eds. John Libbey Eurotext, Paris 1990, 517-519.

[9]   Suzuki F, Brutkiewicz RR, Pollard RB. Co-operation of lymphokine(s) and macrophages in expression of anticancer activity of carboxyethyl germanium sesquioxide (Ge-132). Anticancer Research 1986, 6, 177-182.

[10]   Tanaka N, Ohida J, Ono M, Yoshiwara H, Beika T, Terasawa A, Yamada J, Morioka S, Mannami T, Orita K,] Augmentation of NK activity in peripheral blood lymphocyte in cancer patients by intermittent Ge-132 administration. Gan To Kagaku Ryoho 1984, 11, 1303-1306.

[11]   Funkajawa H, Ohoshi Y, Sekiyama S, Hoshi H, Abe M, Takahashi M, Sato T. Multidisciplinary treatment of head and neck cancer using BCG, OK-432 and GE-132 as biologic response modifiers. Head & Neck 1994, 16(1), 30-38.

[12]   Hill BT, Whatley SA, Bellamy AS, Jenkins LY, Whelan RD. Cytotoxic effects and biological activity of 2-aza-8-germanspiro-[4,5]-decane-2-propanamine-8,8-diethyl-N,N-dimethyl dichloride (NSC 192965; Spirogermanium) in vitro. Cancer Research 1982, 42(7), 2852-2856.

[13]   Slavik M, Blanc O, Davis J. Spirogermanium: a new investigational drug of novel structure and lack of bone marrow toxicity. Investigational New Drugs 1983, 1(3), 225-234.

[14]   Yang SJ, Rafla S. Effect of Spirogermanium on V79 Chinese hamster cells. American Journal of Clinical Oncology 1983, 6, 331-337.

[15]   Mirabelli CK, Badger AM, Sung CP. Pharmacological activities of spirogermanium and other structurally related azaspiranes: effects on tumor cell and macrophage functions. Anticancer Drug Design 1989, 3(4), 231-242.

[16]   Grzybek J. Biological activity of Sanumgerman in allium test. In: 1st Int. Conf. On Germanium, Hanover, Lekim and Samochowiec (eds) October 1984, Semmelwies—Verlag. 1985.

[17]   Kohimunzer S. The allium test as a tool in search for potential oncostatics. In 1st Int. Conf. On Germanium, Hanover, Lekim and Samochowiec (eds). October 1984, Semnelweis Verlag. 1985.

[18] Hill B, Whatley SA, Bellemy AS, Jenkins LH, Whelan RD. Cytotoxic effects and biological activities of NSC-192965; Spirogermanium in vitro. Cancer Research 1982, 42, 2852-2856.

[19] Bespalov VG, Davydov VV, Limarenko Alu, Slepian LI, Aleksandrov VA. The inhibition of the development of experimental tumors of the cervix uteri and vagina by using tinctures of the cultured-cell biomass of the ginseng root and its germanium-selective stocks. Bulletin of Experimental Biology and Medicine 1993, HHG(1), 534-536.

[20] Kopf-Maier P. Cytostatic non-platinum metal complexes: new perspectives for the treatment of cancer. Naturwisseneschaften 1987, 74(8), 374-382.

[21] Brodbeck J. Germanium in biological systems. In 1St Int. Conf. On Germanium, Hanover, October 1984, Lekim and Samochowiec (eds). Semnelweis Verlag. 1985.

[22] Lekim D, Kehlbeck H. The biological activity of germanium. In 1St Int. Conf. On Germanium, Hanover, October 1984, Lekim and Samochowiec (eds). Semnelweis Verlag. 1985.

[23] Schein PS, Slavik M, Smythe T, Hoth D, Smith F, Macdonald JS, Woolley PV. Phase I clinical trial of spirogermanium. Cancer Treatment Reports 1980, 64(10-11), 1051-1056.

[24] Suzuki F. Suppression of tumor growth by peritoneal macrophages isolated from mice treated with carboxyethylgermanium sesquioxide (Ge-132)]. Gan To Kagaku Ryoho 1985, 12(11), 2122-2128.

[25] Suzuki F. Ability of sera from mice treated with Ge-132, an organo-germanium compound, to inhibit experimental murine ascites tumors. Gan To Kagaku Ryoho 1985, 12(12), 2314-2321.

[26] Aso H, Shibuya E, Suzuki F, Nakamura T, Inoue H, Ebina T, Ishida N. Antitumor effect in mice of an organic germanium compound (Ge-132) when different administration methods are used. Gan To Kagaku Ryoho 1985, 12(12), 2345-2351.

[27] Kobayashi H, Komuro T, Furue H. Effect of combination immunochemotherapy with an organogermanium compound, Ge-132, and antitumor agents on C57BL/6 mice bearing Lewis lung carcinoma (3LL). Gan To Kagaku Ryoho 1986, 13(8), 2588-2593.

[28] Suzuki F. Antitumor mechanisms of carboxymethyl-germanium sesquioxide (Ge-132) in mice bearing Ehrlich ascites tumors. Gan To Kagaku Ryoho 1987, 14(1), 127-134.

[29] Kopf-Maier P, Janiak C, Schumann H. Antitumor properties of organometallic metallocene complexes of tin and germanium. Journal of Cancer Research and Clinical Oncology 1988, 114(5), 502-506.

[30] Sato I, Nishimura T, Kakimoto N, Suzuki H, Tanaka N. Prevention of pulmonary metastasis of Lewis lung carcinoma and activation of murine macrophages by a novel organic germanium compound, PCAGeS. Journal of Biological Response Modifiers 1988, 7(1), 1-5.

[31] Jao SW, Lee W, Ho YS. Effect of germanium on 1,2-dimethylhydrazine-induced intestinal cancer in rats. Diseases of the Colon & Rectum 1990, 33(2), 99-104.

[32] Jang JJ, Cho KJ, Lee YS, Bae JH. Modifying responses of allyl sulfide, indole-3carbinol and germanium in a rat multi-organ carcinogenesis model. Carcinogenesis 1991, 12(4), 691-695.

[33] Kobayashi H, Aso H, Ishida N, Maeda H, Schmitt DA, Pollard RB, Suzuki F. Preventive effect of a synthetic immunomodulator, 2-carboxylgermanium sesquioxide on the generation of suppressor microphages in mice immunized with allogeneic lymphocytes. Immunopharmacology and Immunotoxicology 1992, 14(4), 841-864.

[34] Kuwabara M. Immunothermotherapy and related TNS induction in mice. Journal of Veterinary Medical Science 1993, 55(3), 471-473.

[35] Nakada Y, Kosaka T, Kuwabara M, Tanaka S, Sato K, Koide F. Effects of 2-carboxythylgermanium sesquioxide (Ge-132) as an immunological modifier of postsurgical immunosuppression in dogs. Journal of Veterinary Medical Science 1993, 55(5), 95-99.

[36] Bespalov VG, Davydov VV, Limarenko AIu, Slepian LI, Aleksandrov VA. The inhibition of the development of experimental tumors of the cervix uteri and vagina by suing tinctures of the cultured-cell biomass of the ginseng root and its germanium selective stocks.

Bulletin of Experimental Biology and Medicine 1993, 116(11), 534-536.

[37]   Chen F, Zhang Q. Inhibitive effects of spirulina on aberrant crypts in colon induced by dimethylhydrazine. Chung Hua Yu Fang I Hsueh Tsa Chih 1995, 29(1), 13-17.

[38]   Ming X, Yin H, Zhu Z. Effect of dietary selenium and germanium on the precancerous lesion in rat glandular stomach induced by N-methyl-N'-nitro-N-nitrosoguanidine. Chung Hua Wai Ko Tsa Chih 1996, 34(4), 221-223.

[39]   Ishiwata Y, Yokochi S, Mashimoto H, Ninomiya F, Suzuki T. Protection against concanavalin A-induced murine liver injury by the organic germanium compound, propagermanium. Scandanavian Journal of Immunology 1998, 48(6), 605-614.

[40]   Yokochi S, Ishiwata Y, Hashimoto H, Ninomiya F, Suzuki T. Hepatoprotective effect of propagerrnanium on Corynebacterium parvum and lipopolysaccharide-induced liver injury in mice. Scandanavian Journal of Immunology 1998, 48(2), 183-191.

[41]   Goodman S. Therapeutic effects of organic germanium. Medical Hypotheses 1988, 26(3), 207-215.

[42]   Mizushima M, Satoh H, Miyao K. Some pharmacological end clinical aspects of a novel organic germanium compound Ge-132 In: Ist Int. Conf. On germanium, Hanover, Lekim and Samochowiec (eds). October 1984, Semmelwies-Verlag, 1985.

[43]   Trope C, Mattsson W, Gynning I, Johnsson JE, Sigurdsson K, Orbert B. Phase II study of spirogermanium in advanced ovarian malignancy. Cancer Treatment Reports 1981, 65(1-2), 119-120.

[44]   Slavik M, Blanc O, Davis J. Spirogermanium: a new investigational drug of novel structure and lack of bone marrow toxicity. Investigational New Drugs 1983, 1(3), 225-234.

[45]   Bui NB, Chauvergne J, Brunet R, Richaud P, Hoerni B, Lagarde C, Le Guillou M. Metastatic cancer of the prostate: phase II study of spirogermanium. Bulletin du Cancer 1986, 73(1), 65-67.

[46]   Ettinger DS, Finkelstein DM, Donehower RC Chang AYC, Green M, Blum R, Hahn RG, Ruckdeschel JC. Phase II study of N-methylformamide, spirogermanium, and 4-demethoxydaunorubicin in the treatment of non-small cell lung

cancer (EST 3583): an Eastern Cooperative Oncology Group. Medical and Pediatric Oncology 1989, 17(3), 197-201.

[47]   Mainwaring MG, Poor C, Zander DS, Harman E. Complete remission of pulmonar spindle cell carcinoma after treatment with oral germanium sesquioxide. Chest 2000, 117(2), 591-593.

[48]   Badawi AM. and Hafiz AA. Synthesis and immunomodulatory activity of some novel amino acid germinates. Metal Ions in Biology and Medicine 2004, 8, 66-73.

[49]   Badawi AM. Metallated amino acid formulations for immunotherapy against hepatitis, cancer and H/V diseases. Egyptian Patent Application No. 2007030129 dated 13/03/2007.

[50]   Morsy SM, Badawi AM, Jajte JM. Biological activity of some novel cationic germanium and titanium metal based surfactants. Tenside Surfactants Detergents 2009, 46(1), 18-23.

[51]

The Role of Selenium in the Chemoprevention of Carcinogenesis

[1]Professor Abdelfattah M. Badawi and
[1]Professor Sahar M. Ahmed

[1]Professor, Egyptian Petroleum Research Institute,
Nasr City, Cairo, Egypt.

Abstract

2,4,6-Trinitrotoluene (TNT) and petroleum products are the most commonly used chemicals for industrial applications and their exposure occurs occupationally during production. The presence of mutagenic compounds in the urine of workers exposed to TNT has been confirmed. It has been reported that TNT exposed munitions workers in China showed a statistically significant increase in the rate of liver cancer. The association between producing TNT and associated disorders and chemoprevention or anti-carcinogenesis is insufficiently recognized in developing countries. Data from a sequential animal model of experimental hepatocarinogenesis showed that sodium selenite is able to reduce the risk for cancer development in liver. Several selenoprotein genes may be involved with the selenium anticancer effect mechanism. Clinic studies involving more recently studies in humans strongly support the protective role of selenium against various types of cancer. The beneficial effects of selenium studies against carcinogenesis should be extended as a prophylaxis for workers exposed to TNT and petroleum products. Recent studies show that nano-sized selenium (nano-Se) can serve as a potential chemopreventative agent with reduced risk of Se toxicity.

Selenium inhibits chemical carcinogenesis

Selenium compounds have been frequently used as an inhibitors of chemical carcinogenesis induced by dimethylbenz(a)anthracene (DMBA). [1-3] Sodium selenite inhibited aryl hydrocarbon hydroxylase (AHH) activity to a maximum of ≈ 70 % and suppressed the overall metabolism of benzo[a]pyrene. [4] Compared to the sulfur structural analogs, selenium compounds are much more active in cancer prevention and may have a multimodal mechanism in preventing cellular transformation as well as in delaying or inhibiting the expression of malignancy after DMBA exposure. [5] Intake of vegetables, selenium and particularly citrus fruit protects the renal VHL gene from mutation insults. [6]

Selenium in cancer chemoprevention

Sugie et al. [7] have reported that dietary organoselenium compounds induce enzymes that hydroxylate or oxidize the carcinogens and decreases DNA alkylation. Previous studies in animals and humans have shown that selenium compounds can prevent cancer development. The association between production of TNT and associated disorders and chemoprevention or anticarcenogenesis is insufficiently recognized in developing countries. Data from a sequential animal model of experimental hepatocarcinogenesis showed that sodium selenite is able to reduce the risk for cancer development in liver. [8] The mammalian genome encodes 25 selenoprotein genes, each containing one or more molecules of selenium in the form of selenocysteine. There is evidence that several selenoprotein genes may be involved with the mechanism by which selenium provides its anticancer effect. [9] Data on the differential expression patterns reported for selenoprotein genes in tumors versus normal tissue support their role in chemoprevention by selenium. Converging data from epidemiological, ecological, and clinical studies have shown that selenium can decrease the risk of some types of human cancers. Inducing apoptosis is considered an important cellular event that can account for the cancer preventive effect of selenium. [10]

Selenium (Se) compounds are well known to inhibit cell proliferation and induce cell death in human cancer cells. Respective chemical forms of Se are intracellularly metabolized via complicated pathways that target distinct molecules and exhibit varying degrees of anticarcinogenicity in different cancer types. However, the precise mechanisms by which Se activates apoptosis remain poorly understood. The effects of Se compounds, Se-methylselenocysteine (MSC), selenomethionine (SeMet) and selenite on cell proliferation, apoptosis and its pathway in established human carcinoma cell lines (HSC-3, -4, A549, and MCF-7) were investigated. Cancer cells were treated with each Se compound during different periods. Cell apoptosis, caspase activity and endoplasmic reticulum (ER) stress markers were analyzed by flow cytometric or immunoblotting analysis respectively. [11] Epidemiological evidence in humans suggests a role for selenium in reducing cancer incidence and mortality. The ability of selenium dioxide (SeO_2) to enhance lymphocyte progression through the cell cycle in patients with advanced (stage IV) cancer has been demonstrated. Ten patients (mean age 51.9 years, range: 32-74, M/F ratio 3/7) with tumors at different sites were included in the study. The addition of SeO_2 into the culture (1.5 microM) significantly enhanced the progression into the S phase of peripheral blood mononuclear cells (PBMCs) isolated from cancer patients, whilst no significant effect was observed on PBMCs isolated from controls. Reactive oxygen species (ROS) levels were significantly higher, whereas glutathione peroxidase (GPx) activity was significantly lower in cancer patients than controls. Serum levels of IL-6 and TNF alpha were significantly higher in cancer patients than controls. [12] In 2010, there was much research carried out on selenium as a chemoprotective anticancer agent. [13-22]

Occupational cancers

The number of industrial chemicals to which workers are exposed has increased particularly in developing countries. Occupational cancers are now a serious concern in developing countries where exposure levels to hazardous chemicals considerably exceeds regulatory levels established in industrialized countries. An example of an industrialized application is TNT exposure which occurs occupationally during production for filling shells, grenades and demolition bombs. TNT is a contaminant in at least 20 of the U.S. Environmental Protection Agency's (U.S. EPA) National Priorities list sites. [23]

TNT-exposed munitions workers

The presence of mutagenic compounds in the urine of workers exposed to TNT has been confirmed. [24] In a case of chronic occupational exposure to TNT, a 61-year-old man died of hepatocellular carcinoma. [25] A preliminary study of a German population living near the sites of two world war II munitions plants indicated an association between increased rates of some types of leukemia and living in a town near TNT waste from these plants. [26] The study showed increased risk of acute myelogenous leukemia (AML) for adult males and females living near the former explosive plants when compared with adults in a neighboring country. [27] TNT-exposed munitions workers in China reported a statistically significant increase in the rate of liver cancer. [28] Occupational exposure to TNT has caused liver toxicity and related mortality. There are also some case reports of liver cancer from occupational exposure, as well as leukemia. [29] Several lines of evidence suggest that TNT may act through a genotoxic mechanism. One study that looked at gene expression changes in a human hepatoma cell line was uninformative for this purpose, due to severe cytotoxicity making analysis impossible. [30] Human populations exposed to TNT have been inadequately studied with regard to carcinogenicity. [31] Recent results indicated the potential of exposure to dinitrotoluenes (by products of TNT production) leading to increased risk induction of cytotoxic, proteotoxic (HSP 70) and genotoxic (GADD 45/153) proteins in human liver carcinoma (Hep G_2) cells. [31]

2,4,6-Trinitrotoluene (TNT) is an important occupational and environmental pollutant. In TNT-exposed humans, notable toxic manifestations have included aplastic anaemia, toxic hepatitis, cataracts, hepatomegaly and liver cancer. [32]. In factory workers exposed to dinitrotoluenes (DNTs, byproducts of the explosive TNT), a link has been made to many adverse health effects. An association between DNT exposure and increased risk of hepatocellular carcinomas and subcutaneous tumors in rats, as well as renal tumors in mice, has been established. To evaluate the cellular and molecular responses of human liver carcinoma cells following exposure to 2,4-DNT and 2,6-DNT, cytotoxicity was evaluated using the MTT assay. Upon 48 hrs of exposure, LC50 values of 245 +/- 14.724 microg/mL and 300 +/- 5.92 microg/mL were recorded for 2,6-DNT and 2,4-DNT respectively. This indicates that both DNTs are moderately toxic and 2,6-DNT is slightly more toxic to HepG2 cells than 2,4-DNT [33]. Nitrotoluenes, such as 2-nitrotoluene and 2,4-dinitrotoluene are carcinogenic in animal experiments. Humans are exposed to such chemicals in the workplace and in the environment. It is therefore important to develop methods to biomonitor people exposed to nitrotoluenes to prevent the potential harmful effects. [34]. In humans exposed to TNT, the formation of hemoglobin adducts of the amino-dinitrotoluenes is in general concordant with the ratio of urinary excretion. The variations in quantities of excreted metabolites among the different occupational cohorts studied are likely explained by the different routes of exposure to TNT including dermal uptake. Most studies show that urinary excretion of the amino-dinitrotoluenes (4-amino-dinitrotoluene plus 2-amino-dinitrotoluene) in a range of 1 to 10 mg L^{-1} (5-50 microM) are not uncommon for instance in persons employed with the disposal of military waste. [35] Several epidemiological studies and animal experiments showed that 2,4,6-trinitrotoluene induced reproductive system toxicity. Oxidative DNA damage to the testis will play a role in reproductive toxicity induced by TNT and other nitroaromatic compounds. [36] An investigation into the occupational health risk level of workers exposed to 2,4,6-trinitrotoluene in the arms industry was carried out. This was done to provide a basis for revising the standards of diagnosis for chronic TNT poisoning and making protective measures for workers. The retrospective study about the morbidity of total malignant tumor was taken on the male workers exposed to TNT over one year from eight military factories during 1970 to 1995. The morbidity of total malignant tumor in male TNT exposed workers were markedly higher than that of controls and the relative risk (RR) was 2.32. This result was compared to the total malignant tumor mortality of male populations in large and medium cities in 1973 to 1975 and 1990 to 1992. The standardized mortality ratio (SMR) were 71.8 and 179.6 respectively. The CI of 99% was 71.8-144.2, indicating that the morbidity of malignant tumor of male workers exposed to TNT was higher than that of normal populations. Liver cancer morbidity was 31.91% of the total malignant tumor and its mortality was 3.97 times of the controls. [37] Recently reported by Tchounwou et al [38] was the fact that transcriptional responses associated with 2,4,6-trinitrotoluene and two of its byproducts, 2,4- and 2,6-dinitotoluenes, to 13 different recombinant cell lines generated from human liver carcinoma cells (HepG2) by creating stable transfectants of mammalian promoter chloramphenicol acetyl transferase (CAT) gene fusions.

Selenium as a potent protective nutrient

Selenium in the form of selenomethionine (8 ppm) in drinking water daily has been found to be highly effective in reducing cancer incidence in male rats fed 2-acetylaminofluorine (0.05%) in the basal diet for 16 weeks. [39] Epidemiological studies indicated an association between low nutritional selenium status and increased risks of carcinogenesis in various sites of the body. [40] Selenium provided via drinking water for male rats has a significant intestinal cancer prevention effect in the presence of a high dose of 1,2-dimethyhydrazine (20mg/Kg x 20 weeks) and the cancer therapeutic effect of selenium was double protective in this animal model. [41] Evidence is emerging that at least in the case of cancer, the antitumorigenic effect of selenium supplementation arises at least in part from enhanced production of specific selenium containing metabolites, not just from maximal expression of selenoenzymes. A number of novel selenium based compounds which target specific aspects of selenium metabolism are under development and among them are anticancer organoselenium compounds which reduce tissue damage. [42] Many studies in the last several years have shown that selenium is a potent protective nutrient for some forms of cancer. The Arizona Cancer Center posted a selenium fact sheet listing the major functions of selenium in the body. [43] These functions are as follows:

- Selenium is present in the active site of many enzymes including thioredoxin reductase, which catalyzes oxidation-reduction reactions. The reactions may encourage cancerous cells to undergo apoptosis.
- Selenium is a component of the antioxidant enzyme glutathione peroxidase.
- Selenium improves the immune system's ability to respond to infection.
- Selenium causes the formation of natural killer cells.
- P450 enzymes in the liver may be induced by selenium, leading to detoxification of some carcinogenic molecules.
- Selenium inhibits prostaglandins that cause inflammation.
- Selenium can decrease the rate of tumor growth.

Selenium in cancer chemoprevention

Studies examining the relationship between the intake of dietary selenium and the risk of various cancers have shown that low selenium intake is associated with higher cancer rates, including liver cancer. These studies show that dietary organoselenium compounds induce enzymes that hydroxylate or oxidize the carcinogens and decreases DNA alkylation. [44] Previous studies in animals and humans have shown that selenium compounds can prevent cancer development. The association between production of TNT and associated disorders and chemoprevention or anticarcenogenesis is insufficiently recognized by developing countries. Data from a sequential animal model of experimental hepatocarcinogenesis showed that sodium selenite is able to reduce the risk for cancer development in liver. [45] The mammalian genome encodes 25 selenoprotein genes, each contains one or more molecules of selenium in the form of selenocysteine. There is evidence that several selenoprotein genes may be involved with the mechanism by which selenium provides its anticancer effect. [46] Data on the differential expression patterns reported for selenoprotein genes in tumors versus normal tissue support their role in chemoprevention by selenium. Converging data from epidemiological, ecological, and clinical studies have shown that selenium can decrease the risk of some types of human cancers. Inducing apoptosis is considered an important cellular event that can account for the cancer preventive effect of selenium. [47]

Selenium compounds are well known to inhibit cell proliferation and induce cell death in human cancer cells. Respective chemical forms of Se are intracellularly metabolized via complicated pathways which target distinct molecules and exhibit varying degrees of anti-carcinogenicity in different cancer types. However, the precise mechanisms by which Se activates apoptosis remain poorly understood. The effects of Se compounds, Se-methylselenocysteine (MSC), selenomethionine (SeMet) and selenite on cell proliferation, apoptosis and its pathway in established for human carcinoma cell lines (HSC-3, -4, A549, and MCF-7) that were investigated. Cancer cells were treated with each Se compound during different periods. Cell apoptosis, caspase activity and ER stress markers were analyzed by flow cytometric or immunoblotting analysis, respectively. [48]

Basic research and clinical studies involving animal models and more recently studies in humans strongly support the protective role of selenium against various types of cancer. The protective action of selenium involves a combination of various mechanisms and the most important ones are (a) the protective role of selenoproteins/selenoenzymes, (b) the reduction of oxidative stress, (c) the inhibition of DNA adduct formation and (d) the cell cycle arrest. [49] The Nutritional Prevention of Cancer (NPC) study randomized 1,312 high-risk dermatology patients to 200 ug/day of selenium in selenized yeast. This treatment decreased total skin cancer incidence by a statistically significant 25%. [50] The beneficial effect of "Factor D" which is a combination of 50 ug selenium, 30 mg vitamin E and 15mg beta carotene on cancer mortality was still evident up to 10 years after the cessation of supplementation by 29,584 adult participant in Linxian, China from 1991 to 2001. [51]

Selenium is a constituent of the small group of selenocysteine containing selenoproteins and elicits important structural and enzymatic functions. Selenium deficiency has been linked to increased infection risk and adverse mood states. Se has been shown to possess cancer-preventive and cytoprotective activities in both animal models and humans. It is well established that Se has a key role in redox regulation and antioxidant function and hence in membrane integrity, energy metabolism and protection against DNA damage. Recent clinical trials have shown the importance of selenium in clinical oncology. Our own clinical study involving 48 patients suggested that selenium has a positive effect on radiation-associated secondary lymphedema in patients with limb edemas, as well those as in the head and neck region, including endolaryngeal edema. Another randomized phase III study of our group was performed to examine the cytoprotective properties of selenium in radiation oncology. [52]

Micronutrient deficiency disorder (MDD) is considered an order of magnitude because of constant exposure to a millieu that promotes DNA damage. [53] Selenium is now better known as an anticarcinogen and several seleno compounds inhibit or retard carcinogenesis. Wallace et al. [54] have investigated the association between toe nail selenium concentrations and bladder cancer risk in a population based case control study in New Hampshire. Emerging evidence indicated a potential role of selenium in the prevention of several types of cancer including bladder cancer.

Effect of selenium on mutagenesis and carcinogensis induced by N-methyl-N-nitro-N-nitrosoguanidine

The effect N-methyl-N-nitro-N-nitrosoguanidine (MNNG), another carcinogen might be similar to the effect of TNT. Dietary selenenium showed inhibitory effects on carcinogenesis in rat glandular stomach induced by MNNG. [55] Sodium selenite when combined with the carcinogen MNNG showed an anticancer effect. [56] Sodium selenite also showed protection from the damage of genetic materials induced by

MNNG. [57] Selenium also has a protective effect on killing mutations induced by MNNG in E. coli. [58] Dietary selenium and germanium have a preventive effect on the precarcinoma lesions in the rat glandular stomach induced by MNNG. [59]

Selenium against tumors

Proposed mechanisms for selenium anticancer action are antioxidant protection, enhanced carcinogen detoxification and enhanced immune surveillance, modulation of cell proliferation, inhibition of human cell invasion and inhibition of angiogenesis. [60] The anticarcinogenic effects of selenium compounds constitute intermediate mechanisms with several underlying chemical/biochemical mechanisms such as redox cycling, alteration of protein thiol redox status and methionine mimicry. [61] Diphenyl selenide proved to be a chemopreventive agent against N-nitroso-methylurea (NMU) induced mammary carcinogenesis in female Wister rats. [62] Dihexyl diselenide has been recorded as a positive treatment toward the prevention of cutaneous and subcutaneous cancer for both male and female subjects. [63] High levels of selenium compounds can effectively inhibit hepatocarcingenesis in transgenic mice. [64] Sodium sulfite reacted with elemental selenium to yield nanoparticle size selenosulfate. In vitro sodium selenosulfate killed Hept G_2 in a dose-dependent fashion and showed a consistent cytotoxic effect against 3 kinds of leukemia cells. [65] Recently reported exposure of human leukemia NB_4 cells to increasing concentrations of selenite switches the signaling from pro-survival to pro-apoptosis. [66] Also, organic derivatives of selenium showed differential sensitivity towards various tumor derived cell types to apoptosis. [67] Selenium at the nano size (nano-Se) level possessed equal efficacy in increasing the activities of each of glutathione peroxidase, thioredoxin reductase and glutathione-S-transferase but had a much lower level of toxicity as indicated by the median lethal dose, acute liver injury, survival rate and short-term toxicity. The results suggest that nano-Se can serve as a potential chemopreventive agent with reduced risk of Se toxicity. [68]

Combination of antioxidants, vitamins and minerals could reduce the risk of skin cancers (SC). A study was performed within the framework of the Supplementation in Vitamins and Mineral Antioxidants study. This was a randomized, double-blinded, placebo controlled, primary prevention trial designed at testing the efficacy of nutritional doses (120 mg vitamin C, 30 mg vitamin E, 6 mg beta-carotene, 100 mg selenium and 20 mg zinc) of antioxidants in reducing incidence of cancer and ischemic heart disease in the general population. [69] High doses of antioxidant supplements may be deleterious in high risk subjects without any clinical symptoms in whom the initial phase of cancer development has already started. [70] There was a marked statistically significant reduction in the rate of prostate cancer for men receiving the supplements. [71] However, a significant interaction between sex and group effects on cancer incidence was found (P = 0.004). After 7.5 years, low-dose antioxidant supplementation lowered total cancer incidence and all-cause mortality in men but not in women. Supplementation may be effective in men only because of their lower baseline status of certain antioxidants, especially of beta carotene. [72]

Potential Antitumor Selenium Metal-Based Surfactants

Badawi et al. [73] recently investigated some novel metal based cationic hydrogen selenite surfactants. Cobalt based surface active hydrogen selenite showed the highest effect on human tumor cell lines. IC-50 for H_{460} (lung cancer), MCF_2 (breast cancer), $HEPG_2$ (liver caner) and HCT_{116} (colon carcinoma) recorded: 1.1, 9.6, 8.6 and 8.66 µg/ml. The antitumor activity might be attributed to lipid peroxidation, DNA, damage and/or reduction of bioenergetic status of tumor tissues.

Conclusion

There is evidence of carcinogenicity arising from working with TNT. Petroleum products also have the potential to induce cytotoxic, proteotoxic, genotoxic and stress gene effects in human liver carcinoma cells. The beneficial effects of selenium studies against carcinogenesis should be extended as a prophylaxis for TNT and petroleum industry exposed workers who have an increased risk of cancer that may well result from increased exposure to TNT and the petroleum industry. Sodium selenite is able to reduce the cancer development in the liver. Cobalt based hydrogen selenite surfactants showed significant potential antitumor activity against broad spectrum lung, breast, liver and colon cancers and this study should be extended to evolve effective chemotherapy for cancer patients.

References

[1]   Ip C and Sinha D. Anticarcinogenic effect of selenium in rats treated with dimethylbenz(ii)anthracene and fed different levels and types of fat. Carcinogenesis 1981, 2, 435-438.

[2]   Medina D, Shepherd F. Selenium-mediated inhibition of 7,12-dimethylbenz[a]anthracene-induced mouse mammary tumorigenesis. Carcinogenesis 1981, 2(5), 451-455.

[3]   Thompson HJ, Meeker LD, Becci PJ, Kokoska S. Effect of short-term feeding of sodium selenite on 7,12-dimethylbenz(a) anthracene-induced mammary carcinogenesis in the rat. Cancer Research 1982, 42, 4954-4958.

[4]   Lin WS, Scrimshaw C, Kapoor M. Selenium suppresses the metabolism of benzo[a]pyrene by rat-liver extracts, and exerts a dual effect on its mutagenicity. Xenobiotica 1984, 14, 893-902.

[5]   Ip C, Ganther HE. Comparison of selenium and sulfur analogs in cancer prevention. Carcinogenesis 1992, 13, 1167-1170.

[6]   El-Bayoumy K and Sinha R. Mechanisms of mammary cancer chemoprevention by organoselenium compounds. Mutation Research 2004, 551, 181-197.

[7]   Sugie T and Tanaka S. El-Bayoumy K. Chemoprevention of carcinogenesis by organoselenium compounds. Journal of Health Science 2000, 46(6), 422-226.

[8]   Bjorkhem L, Torndal U, Eken S. Selenium prevents tumor development in a rat model for chemical carcinogenesis. Carcinogenesis 2005, 20(1), 125-131.

[9]   Diwadkar-Navsariwala V and Diamond AM. Recent advances in nutritional science. The link between selenium and chemoprevention: A case for selenoproteins. Journal of Nutrition 2004, 134, 2899-2902.

[10] Rikiishi H. Apoptotic cellular events for selenium compounds involved in cancer prevention Journal of Bioengineering and Biomedical Science 2008, 39(1), 91-98.

[11] Suzuki M, Endo M, Shinohara F, Echigo S, Rikiishi H. Differential apoptotic response of human cancer cells to organoselenium compounds. Cancer Chemotherapy and Pharmacology 2010, 66, 475-484.

[12] Rinaldi A, Journal of Experimental Therapeutics and Oncology 2004, 4(1), 69-78.

[13] Novotny L, Rauko P, Kombian S, Edafiogho I. Neoplasma. 2010, 57(5), 383-391.

[14] Carlson BA, Yoo MH, Shrimali RK, Irons R, Gladyshev VN, Hatfield DL, Park JM, Proceedings of the Nutrition Society 2010, 69(3), 300-310.

[15] Roth MJ, Katki HA, Wei WQ, Qiao YL, Bagni R, Wang GQ, Whitby D, Dong ZW, Gail MH, Limburg PJ, Giffen CA, Taylor PR, Dawsey SM. Cancer Prevention Research 2010, 3(7), 810-817.

[16] Büntzel J, Riesenbeck D, Glatzel M, Berndt-Skorka R, Riedel T, Mücke R, Kisters K, Schönekaes KG, Schäfer U, Bruns F, Micke O. Anticancer Research 2010, 30(5), 1829-1832.

[17] Sinha R, Sinha I, Facompre N, Russell S, Somiari RI, Richie JP, El-Bayoumy K. Cancer Epidemiology Biomarkers & Prevention 2010, 19(9), 2332-2340.

[18] Zhang J, Wang L, Anderson L, Witthuhn B, Xu Y, Lü J. Cancer Prevention Research 2010, 3(8), 994-1006.

[19] Stratton MS, Algotar AM, Ranger-Moore J, Stratton SP, Slate EH, Hsu CH, Thompson PA, Clark LC, Ahmann FR. Cancer Prevention Research 2010, 3(8), 1035-1043.

[20] Jiang L, Yang KH, Tian JH, Guan QL, Yao N, Cao N, Mi DH, Wu J, Ma B, Yang SH. Nutrition and Cancer 2010, 62(6), 719-727.

[21] Zachara BA, Gromadzinska J, Palus J, Zbrog Z, Swiech R, Twardowska E, Wasowicz W. The effect of selenium supplementation in the prevention of DNA damage in white blood cells of hemodialyzed patients: A pilot study. Biological Trace Element Research 2010, 142, 274-283.

[22] Poarco N, Mantos E, Vainio H, Kovinas M. Occupational cancers in developing countries IARC Scientific Publications 1994, 129

[23] Toxicological profile for 2,4,6-trinitrotoluene. ASTSDR., U.S. Department Of Health And Human Sevices. Public Health Service. Agency for Toxic Substances And Disease Registery (ATSDR, 1995).

[24] Ahlborg Jr G, Einisto P, Sorsa M. Mutagenic activity and metabolites in the urine of workers exposed to TNT. British Journal of Industrial Medicine 1988, 45(5) 353-358.

[25] Garfinkel D, Sidi Y, Steier M. Liver cirrhosis and hepatocellular carcinoma after prolonged exposure to TNT: Causal relationship or mere coincidence. Med Intern 1988, 26(41), 287-290.

[26] Kolb G, Becker N, Scheller S. Increased risk of acute myelogenous leukemia (CML) and chronic myelogenous leukemia (CML) in a country of Hesse, Germany. Sozial und Präventivmedizin/Social and Preventive Medicine 1993, 38(4), 190-195.

[27] Kilian P, Skrzypek S, Becker N, Havemann K. Exposure to armament wastes and leukemia: a case-control study within a cluster of AML and CML in Germany Leukemia Research 2001, 25(10), 839-845.

[28] Sabbioni G, Liu Y, Yan H, Sepai O. Hemoglobin adducts, urinary metabolites and health effects in 2,4,6-trinitrotoluene exposed workers. Carcinogenesis 2005, 26(7), 1272-1279.

[29] Yan C, Wang Y, Xia B. The retrospective survey of malignant tumor in weapon workers exposed to TNT. Chin. Journal of Industrial Hygiene and Occupational Diseases 2002, 20, 184-188.

[30] Tchounwou PB, Wilson BA. Ishaque AB, Schneider J. Transcription activation of stress genes and cytotoxicity in human liver carcinoma cells (Hep G2) exposed to 2,4,6-trinitrotoluene, 2,4-dinitrotoluene, and 2,6-dinitrotoluene. Environmental Toxicology 2001, 16 209-216.

[31] Glass KY, Newsome CR, Tchounwou PB. Cytotoxicity and expression of C-fos, HSP 70 and GADD 45/153 proteins in human liver carcinoma (Hep G_2) cells exposed to dinitrotoluenes. International Journal of Environmental Research and Public Health 2005, 2(2), 355-361.

[32]   Sabbioni G, Sepai O, Norppa H, Yan H, Hirvonen A, Zheng Y, Järventaus H, Bäck B, Brooks L, Warren S, Demarini D, Liu Y. Comparison of biomarkers in workers exposed to 2,4,6-trinitrotoluene. Biomarkers 2007, 12(1), 21-37.

[33]   Glass K, Newsome C, Tchounwou P. Cytotoxicity and expression of c-fos, HSP70, and GADD45/153 proteins in human liver carcinoma (HepG2) cells exposed to dinitrotoluenes. International Journal of Environmental Research and Public Health 2005, 2(2), 355-361.

[34]   Sabbioni G, Jones C, Sepai O, Hirvonen A, Norppa H, Järventaus H, Glatt H, Pomplun D, Yan, H, Brooks L, Warren S, Demarini D, Liu Y. Biomarkers of exposure, effect, and susceptibility in workers exposed to nitrotoluenes. Cancer Epidemiology, Biomarkers and Prevention 2006, 15(3) 559-566.

[35]   Bolt H, Degen G, Dorn S, Plöttner S, Harth V. Genotoxicity and potential carcinogenicity of 2,4,6-TNT trinitrotoluene: structural and toxicological considerations. Reviews on Environmental Health 2006, 21(4), 217-228.

[36]   Homma-Takeda S, Hiraku Y, Ohkuma Y, Oikawa S, Murata M, Ogawa K, Iwamuro T, Li S, Sun G, Kumagai Y, Shimojo N, Kawanishi S. 2,4,6-Trinitrotoluene-induced reproductive toxicity via oxidative DNA damage by its metabolite. Free Radical Research 2002, 36(5), 555-566.

[37]   Yan C, Wang Y, Xia B, Li L, Zhang Y, Liu Y. The retrospective survey of malignant tumor in weapon workers exposed to 2,4,6-trinitrotoluene. Zhonghua Lao Dong Wei Sheng Zhi Ye Bing Za Zhi 2002, 20(3), 184-188.

[38]   Tchounwou P, Wilson B, Ishaque A, Schneider J. Transcriptional activation of stress genes and cytotoxicity in human livercarcinoma cells (HepG2) exposed to 2,4,6-trinitrotoluene, 2,dinitrotoluene, and2,6-dinitrotoluene. Environmental Toxicology 2001, 16(3), 209-216.

[39]   Mukherejee B, Sarkar A, Chatterjee M. Biochemical basis of selenomethionine-mediated inhibition during 2-acetylamino-fluorene-induced hepatocarcinogenesis in the rat. European journal of cncer prevention. 1996, 5(6), 455-463.

[40] Badmaev V, Majeed M, Passwater R. Selenium: a quest for better understanding. Alternative Therapies, Health and Medicine 1996, 2(4), 65-67.

[41] Jao SW, Shen KL, Lee W. Effect of selenium on 1,2 dimethylhydrazine-induced intestinal cancer in rats. Diseases of the Colon and Rectum 1996, 89(6), 628-631.

[42] May SW. Selenium-based pharmacological agents: An update. Expert Opinion on Investigational Drugs 2002, 11(9), 1261-1269.

[43] Donaldson MS. Nutrition and Cancer: A review of the evidence of anticancer diet. Nutrition Journal 2004, 3(19), 1-45.

[44] Sugie S,Tanaka T, El-Bayoumy K. Chemoprevention of carcinogenesis by organoselenium compounds. Journal of Health Sciences 2000, 46(6), 422-226.

[45] Bjorkhem L,Torndal U, Eken S. Selenium prevents tumor development in a rat model for chemical carcinogenesis. Carcinogenesis 2005, 20(1), 125-131.

[46] Diwadkar-Navsariwala and V, Diamond AM. Recent advances in nutritional science, The link between selenium and chemoprevention: A case for selenoproteins. Journal of Nutrition 2004, 134, 2899-2902.

[47] Rikiishi H. Apoptotic cellular events for selenium compounds involved in cancer prevention Journal of Bioenergetics and Biomembranes 2007, 39(1), 91-98.

[48] Suzuki M, Endo M, Shinohara F, Echigo S, Rikiishi H. Differential apoptotic response of human cancer cells to organoselenium compounds. Cancer Chemotherapy and Pharmacology 2010, 66(3), 475-484.

[49] Naithani R. Organoselenium in cancer prevention. Mini-Reviews in Medicinal Chemistry 2008, 8(7), 657-668.

[50] Reid ME, Duftield-Lillico AJ, Slate E. The nutrition preventional of cancer. Nutrition and Cancer 2008, 60(2), 155-163.

[51] QiaoYL, Dawsey SM, Kamangar F. Total and cancer mortality after supplementation with vitramins and minerals: Follow-up of the Linxian General Population Nutrition Intervention Trial. Journal of the National Cancer Institute. 2009, 101(7), 507-518.

[52] Micke O, Schomburg L, Buentzel J, Kisters K, Muecke R. Selenium in oncology: from chemistry to clinics. Molecules 2009, 14(10), 3975-3988.

[53] Anetor JI, Anetor GO, Udah DC, Adenya FAA. Chemical carcinogenesis and chemoprevention: scientific priority area in rapidly industrializing developing countries. African Journal of Environmental Science and Technology 2008, 2(7), 150-156.

[54] Wallace K, Kelsey K, Schned A, Morris J, Andrew A, Karagas M. Selenium and risk of bladder cancer: a population-based case-control study. Cancer Prevention Research, 2009, 2(1), 70-73.

[55] Kobayashi M., Kogata M, Yamamura M. Inhibitory effect of dietary selenium on carcinogenesis in rat glandular stomach induced by N-methyl-N'-nitro-N-nitrosoguanidine. Cancer Research 1986, 46(5), 2266-2270.

[56] Chen QG, Gao FZ, Ke Y. Effect of sodium selenite on the chemosomal aberration of V79 cells induced in vitro by MNNG and MNU. Zhonghua Zhoug Liu Za Zhi 1987, 9(1), 33-35.

[57] An J, Chen QG, Gao FZ, Zheng E. Effect of Na_2SeO_3 on the damage of genetic materials induced by MNNG in children's foreskin fibroblasts in vitro. Zhonghua Zhong Liu Za Zhi 1988, 10(3), 180-183.

[58] Sato M, Nunoshiba T, Nishioka H. Protective effects of sodium selenite on killing and mutation by N-methyl-N'-nitro-N-nitrosoguanidine in E. coli. Mutation Research 1991, 250(1-2), 73-77.

[59] Mino X,Yin H, Zhu Z. Effect of dietary selenium and germanium on the precancerous lesion in rat glandular stomach induced by N-methyl-N'-nitro-N-nitrosoguanidine. Zhonghua Wai ke Za Zhi 1996, 34(4), 221-223.

[60] Zeng Hand Combs Jr GF. Selenium as anticancer nutrient: roles in cell proliferation and tumor cell invasion. Journal of Nutritional Biochemistry 2008, 19(1), 1-7.

[61] Jackson MI and Combs Jr GF. Selenium and anticarcinigenesis: underlying mechanisms. Clinical Nutrition & Metabolic Care 2008, 11(6), 718-26.

[62]   Barbosa N and Noguera CW. Diphenyl diselenide supplemenatation delays the development of N-nitroso-N-methylurea-induced mammary tumors. Genotoxicity and Carcinogenecity 2008, 82, 655-663.

[63]   Schrauzer G, Compositions for the treatment of cancer. US. Patent, 7,521,665 (2009).

[64]   Novoselov SV, Calvisi DF, Labunsky VM. Selenoprotein deficiency and high levels of selenium compounds can effectively inhibit hepatocarcinogenesis in transgeneic mice. Oncogene 2005, 24(54), 3003-3011.

[65]   Zhang J, Lu H, Wang X. MSO7116 Sodium selenosulfate synthesis and demonstration of its in vitro cytotoxic activity against Hep G_2, $CaCO_2$, and three kinds of leukemia cells. Biological Trace Element Research 2008, 125(1), 13-21.

[66]   Guan L, Han B, Li J. Exposure of human leukemia NB_4 cells to increasing concentrations of selenite switches the signalining from pro-survival to pro-apoptosis. Annals of Hematology 2009, 88(8), 733-42.

[67]   Jariwalla BJ, Gangapurkar B, Nakamura D. Differential sensitivity of various human tumour—derived cell types to apoptosis by organic derivatives of selenium. British Journal of Nutrition 2009, 101(2), 182-189.

[68]   Zhang J, Wang X, Xu T. Elemental selenium at nano size (Nano-Se) as a potential chemopreventive agent with reduced risk of selenium toxicity: Comparison with Se-methylseleinocysteine in Mice. Toxicological Sciences 2008, 101(1), 22-31.

[69]   Hercberg S, Ezzedine K, Guinot C, Preziosi P, Galan P, Bertrais S, Estaquio C, Briançon S, Favier A, Latreille J, Malvy D. Antioxidant supplementation increases the risk of skin cancers in women but not in men. Journal of Nutrition, 2007, 137(9), 2098-2105.

[70]   Hercberg S. The SU.VI.MAX study, a randomized, placebo-controlled trial on the effects of antioxidant vitamins and minerals on health]. Annales Pharmaceutique Francaises 2006, 64(6), 397-401.

[71]   Meyer F, Galan P, Douville P, Bairati I, Kegle P, Bertrais S, Estaquio C, Hercberg S. Antioxidant vitamin and mineral supplementation and

prostate cancer prevention in the SU.VI.MAX trial. International Journal of Cancer 2005, 116(2), 182-186.

[72]   Hercberg S, Galan P, Preziosi P, Bertrais S, Mennen L, Malvy D, Roussel AM, Favier A, Briançon S. The SU.VI. MAX Study: a randomized, placebo-controlled trial of the health effects of antioxidant vitamins and minerals. Archives of Internal Medicine 2004, 164(21), 2335-2342.

[73]   Badawi AM, Mekawi AM, Mohamed MZ, Khowdairy MM. Surface and antitumor activity of some novel metal-based cationic surfactants. Journal of Cancer Research and Therapeutics 2007, 3(4), 198-206.

The Role of Metal Ions as Protecting Against against Chemical Carcinogenesis

[1]Dr Philippe Collery, [2]Dr Abdelfattah Badawi and [3]Dr Sunali Khanna

[1]Dr, Service de Cancérologie and Centre de Recherche et Développement de Composés Organo Métalliques à Usage Thérapeutique, Polyclinique Maymard, 20200 Bastia, France. [2]ProfessorEgyptian Petroleum Research Institute, Cairo, Egypt and Centre de Recherche et Développement de Composés Organo Métalliques à Usage Thérapeutique, Bastia, France. [3]Professor, Vice President, Indian Academy of Oral Medicine & Radiology, Assistant Professor, Department of Oral Medicine & Radiology, Nair Hospital Dental College, Mumbai-400 008, India

Introduction

Occupational and Environmental Causes of Respiratory Cancers (ICARE):

Occupational causes of respiratory cancers need to be further investigated. The role of occupational exposures in the aetiology of head and neck cancers remains largely unknown and there are still substantial uncertainties for a number of suspected lung carcinogens. The main objective of the study is to examine occupational risk factors for lung and head and neck cancers.

ICARE is a multicenter population based case control study, which includes a group of 2926 lung cancer cases, a group of 2415 head and neck cancer cases and a common control group of 3555 subjects. Incident cases were identified in collaboration with cancer registries in 10 geographical areas. The control group was a random sample of the population of these areas, with distribution by sex and age comparable to cases and a distribution by socioeconomic status comparable to that of the population. Subjects were interviewed face to face using a standardized questionnaire collecting particularly information on tobacco and alcohol consumption, residential history and a detailed description of occupational history. Biological samples were also collected from study subjects. The main occupational exposures of interest were asbestos, man-made mineral fibers, formaldehyde, polycyclic aromatic hydrocarbons, chromium and nickel compounds, arsenic, wood dust, textile dust, solvents, strong acids, cutting fluids, silica, diesel fumes and welding fumes. The complete list of exposures of interest included more than 60 substances. Occupational exposure assessment used several complementary methods: case-by-case evaluation of exposure by experts, development and use of algorithms to assess exposure from the questionnaires and application of job exposure matrices.

The large number of subjects associated with moderate increase in risks and the evaluation of risks associated with infrequent or widely dispersed exposures. It is possible to study joint effects of exposure to different occupational risk factors, to examine the interactions between occupational exposures, tobacco smoking, alcohol drinking, and genetic risk factors and to estimate the proportion of respiratory cancers attributable to occupational exposures in France. In addition, information on many non-occupational risk factors is available, and the study will provide an excellent framework for numerous studies in various fields. [1]

Gallium nitrate for prevention of osteolysis in myeloma

Since osteolysis is a major cause of morbidity in myeloma, we conducted a pilot study to evaluate whether the addition of gallium nitrate to standard antimyeloma treatment could preserve or increase bone mass in patients with osteolytic disease.

Patients stabilized on cytotoxic therapy were randomized to treatment with gallium nitrate for 6 months or to observation only for the first 6 months followed by gallium nitrate treatment during the subsequent 6 months. Gallium nitrate was administered in monthly cycles by daily subcutaneous injections (30 mg/m2/d) for 2 weeks, followed by 2 weeks with no therapy, supplemented by an intravenous infusion (100 mg/m2/d) for 5 days every other month.

Paired 6-month comparisons were available for seven observation periods and 13 gallium nitrate treatment periods. Total body calcium assessed by delayed gamma neutron activation (DGNA) decreased in four of seven patients during observation, but increased in nine of 13 patients during gallium nitrate treatment. The mean difference in total body calcium (TBCa) between the two groups at 6 months was 3%. Median regional bone density assessed by dual photon absorptiometry (DPA) declined by 1.4% in patients under observation (range +6.7% to -18.3%) but was unchanged during gallium nitrate treatment (median change 0%; range -10.5% to +14.4%). The group mean vertebral fracture index assessed by lateral spine X-rays decreased by 27% during observation compared with 2% during gallium nitrate treatment. Mean body height decreased by 0.57 inches in the observation group and 0.06 inches in the gallium nitrate group. Patient self-assessment of bone pain showed that seven of 12 gallium nitrate treated patients rated themselves as experiencing major reductions in bone pain compared with zero of seven patients who were observed. One episode of hypercalcemia occurred in a patient under observation.

Adjuvant treatment with low dose gallium nitrate attenuates the rate of bone loss in myeloma and may be useful for ameliorating the consequences of skeletal morbidity in patients with cancer related osteolysis. [2]

Oral mucositis prevention by gallium-aluminum-arsenide LLL therapy in head-and neck cancer patients undergoing concurrent chemoradiotherapy

Oral mucositis is a major complication of concurrent chemoradiotherapy (CRT) in head and neck cancer patients. Low level laser (LLL) therapy is a promising preventive therapy. We aimed to evaluate the efficacy of LLL therapy to decrease severe oral mucositis and its effect on RT interruptions.

In this randomized, double-blind, Phase III study, patients received either gallium-aluminum-arsenide LLL therapy 2.5 J/cm(2) or placebo laser treatment before each radiation fraction. Eligible patients had to have been diagnosed with squamous cell carcinoma or undifferentiated carcinoma of the oral cavity, pharynx, larynx, or metastases to the neck with an unknown primary site. They were treated with adjuvant or definitive CRT, consisting of conventional RT 60-70 Gy (range, 1.8-2.0 Gy/d, 5 times/wk) and concurrent cisplatin. The primary endpoints were the oral mucositis severity in Weeks 2, 4, and 6 and the number of RT interruptions because of mucositis. The secondary endpoints included patient reported pain scores. To detect a decrease in the incidence of Grade 3 or 4 oral mucositis from 80% to 50%, we planned to enroll 74 patients.

A total of 75 patients were included and 37 patients received preventive LLL therapy. The mean delivered radiation dose was greater in the patients treated with LLL (69.4 vs. 67.9 Gy, p = .03). During CRT, the number of patients diagnosed with Grade 3 or 4 oral mucositis treated with LLL vs placebo was 4 vs 5 (Week 2, p = 1.0), 4 vs 12 (Week 4, p = .08) and 8 vs 9 (Week 6, p = 1.0), respectively. More of the patients treated with placebo had RT interruptions because of mucositis (6 vs. 0, p = .02). No difference was detected between the treatment arms in the incidence of severe pain.

LLL therapy was not effective in reducing severe oral mucositis, although a marginal benefit could not be excluded. It reduced RT interruptions in these head and neck cancer patients, which might translate into improved CRT efficacy. [3]

Zinc in cancer prevention

The essentiality of zinc for humans was discovered 45 years ago. Deficiency of zinc is prevalent world wide in developing countries and may affect nearly 2 billion subjects. The major manifestations of zinc deficiency include growth retardation, hypogonadism in males, cell mediated immune dysfunctions and cognitive impairment. Zinc not only improves cell mediated immune functions but also functions as an antioxidant and anti-inflammatory agent. Oxidative stress and chronic inflammation have been implicated in the development of many cancers. In patients with head and neck cancer, we have shown that nearly 65% of these patients were zinc deficient based on their cellular zinc concentrations. Natural killer (NK) cell activity and IL-2 generation were also affected adversely. Th2 cytokines were not affected. In our patients, zinc status was a better indicator of tumor burden and stage of disease in comparison to the overall nutritional status. Zinc status also correlated with number of hospital admissions and incidences of infections. NF-kappa B is constitutively activated in many cancer cells and this results in activation of anti-apoptotic genes, VEGF, cyclin DI, EGFR, MMP-9 and inflammatory cytokines. Zinc inhibits NF-kappa B via induction of A-20. Thus, zinc supplementation should have beneficial effects on cancer by decreasing angiogenesis and induction of inflammatory cytokines while increasing apoptosis in cancer cells. Based on the above, we recommend further studies and propose that zinc should be utilized in the management and chemoprevention of cancer. [4]

Influence of extraneous supplementation of zinc on prevention of dimethylhydrazine induced colon carcinogenesis

Trace elemental analyses of cancerous tissue is a less explored field of inquiry in cancer research. If the deficiency or excess of a particular trace element can be linked to the cancer, studies can be initiated to see its controlled administration to check the growth of cancer. The present study explored the prophylactic potential of zinc in experimental colon carcinogenesis and also its interaction with other trace metals, which gets altered during the development of colon cancer. Rats were segregated into four groups: 1. normal control, 2. dimethylhydrazine (DMH) treated, 3. zinc treated and 4. DMH+zinc treated. Initiation and induction of colon carcinogenesis was achieved through weekly subcutaneous injections of DMH (30 mg/Kg body weight) dissolved in 1 mM EDTA in normal saline (pH 6.5) for 8 and 16 weeks respectively. Zinc was supplemented at a dose level of 227 mg/L in drinking water for 8 and 16 weeks. The elemental analyses of colonic samples were carried out using Energy Dispersive X-Ray Fluorescence technique (EDXRF). Zinc administration to DMH treated rats significantly decreased the tumor incidence multiplicity with simultaneous decrement in tumor size. EDXRF studies revealed that the concentrations of the elements zinc, chromium, manganese and copper were decreased, whereas the concentration levels of iron were found to be increased in the colon tissues following 8 and 16 weeks of DMH treatment. However, zinc supplementation to DMH treated rats significantly improved the altered levels of elements when compared to DMH treated animals indicating the chemopreventive role of zinc. In conclusion, DMH induced colon carcinogenesis is accompanied by altered trace element profile and zinc has a positive beneficial effect against chemically induced colonic carcinogenesis. [5]

Chemopreventive potential of zinc in experimentally induced colon carcinogenesis

This study was performed to evaluate the efficacy of zinc treatment on the colonic antioxidant defense system and histo-architecture in

1,2-dimethylhydrazine (DMH) induced colon carcinogenesis in male Sprague-Dawley rats. The rats were segregated into four groups: 1. normal control, 2. DMH treated, 3. zinc treated and 4. DMH+zinc treated. Colon carcinogenesis was induced through weekly subcutaneous injections of DMH (30 mg/kg body weight) for 16 weeks. Zinc (in the form of zinc sulphate) was supplemented to rats at a dose level of 227 mg/L in drinking water ad libitum for the entire duration of the study. Increased tumor incidence, tumor size and number of aberrant crypt foci (ACF) were accompanied by a decrease in lipid peroxidation, glutathione-S-transferase, superoxide dismutase (SOD) and catalase. On the contrary, significantly increased levels of reduced glutathione (GSH) and glutathione reductase (GR) were observed in DMH treated rats. Administration of zinc to DMH treated rats significantly decreased the tumor incidence, tumor size and aberrant crypt foci number with simultaneous enhancement of lipid peroxidation, SOD, catalase and glutathione-S-transferase. Further, the levels of GSH and GR were also decreased following zinc supplementation to DMH treated rats. Well differentiated signs of dysplasia were evident in colonic tissue sections by DMH administration alone. However, zinc treatment to DMH treated rats greatly restored normalcy in the colonic histo-architecture, with no apparent signs of neoplasia. EDXRF studies revealed a significant decrease in tissue concentrations of zinc in the colon following DMH treatment, which upon zinc supplementation were recovered to near normal levels. In conclusion, the results of this study suggest that zinc has a positive beneficial effect against chemically induced colonic preneoplastic progression in rats induced by DMH. [6]

Carcinogenesis protection by zinc

This study explored the regulatory role of zinc on the *in vitro* uptake of ^{14}C-glucose and ^{14}C-labeled amino acids and on colonic surface abnormalities after 1,2-dimethylhydrazine (DMH) induced colon carcinogenesis. Rats were segregated into four groups: 1. control, 2. DMH treated, 3. zinc treated and 4. DMH+zinc-treated. Colon carcinogenesis was induced through weekly subcutaneous injections of DMH (30 mg/kg body weight) for 16 weeks. Zinc (in the form of zinc sulfate) was given to rats at a dose level of 227 mg/L in their drinking water. DMH treatment caused a significant decrease in the activities of disaccharidases (sucrase, lactase, and maltase), but a significant increase in the activity of alkaline phosphatase. In vitro uptake of ^{14}C-D-glucose and the amino acids ^{14}C-glycine, ^{14}C-alanine, ^{14}C-lysine and ^{14}C-leucine were significantly higher in the colon of DMH treated rats. Zinc supplementation of DMH treated rats resulted in regulating the altered intestinal enzyme activities and in vitro uptake of ^{14}C-amino acids and ^{14}C-glucose. Scanning electron microscopy revealed drastic alterations in the colon surface morphology after DMH treatment, which restored after zinc supplementation. Our results confirm a beneficial effect of zinc against DMH induced alterations in the colons of rats. [7]

Effect of zinc on immune cells

Although the essentiality of zinc for plants and animals has been known for many decades, the essentiality of zinc for humans was recognized only 40 years ago in the Middle East. The zinc deficient patients had severe immune dysfunctions, inasmuch as they died of intercurrent infections by the time they were 25 years of age. In our studies in an experimental human model of zinc deficiency, we documented decreased serum testosterone level, oligospermia, severe immune dysfunctions mainly affecting T helper cells, hyperammonemia, neurosensory disorders and decreased lean body mass. It appears that zinc deficiency is prevalent in the developing world and as many as two billion subjects may be growth retarded due to zinc deficiency. Besides growth retardation and immune dysfunctions, cognitive impairment due to zinc deficiency also has been reported recently. Our studies in cell culture models showed that the activation of many zinc dependent enzymes and transcription factors were adversely affected due to zinc deficiency. In the HUT-78 (T helper 0 [Th(0)] cell line), we showed that a decrease in gene expression of interleukin-2 (IL-2) and IL-2 receptor alpha(IL-2Ralpha) were due to decreased activation of nuclear factor-kappaB (NF-kappaB) in zinc deficient cells. Decreased NF-kappaB activation in HUT-78 due to zinc deficiency was due to decreased binding of NF-kappaB to DNA, decreased level of NF-kappaB p105 (the precursor of NF-kappaB p50) mRNA, decreased kappaB inhibitory protein (IkappaB) phosphorylation and decreased Ikappa kappa. These effects of zinc were cell specific. Zinc also is an antioxidant and has anti-inflammatory actions. The therapeutic roles of zinc in acute infantile diarrhea, acrodermatitis enteropathica, prevention of blindness in patients with age related macular degeneration and treatment of common cold with zinc have been reported. In HL-60 cells (promyelocytic leukemia cell line), zinc enhances the up-regulation of A20 mRNA, which, via TRAF pathway, decreases NF-kappaB activation, leading to decreased gene expression and generation of tumor necrosis factor-alpha (TNF-alpha), IL-1beta and IL-8. We have reported recently that in both young adults and elderly subjects, zinc supplementation decreased oxidative stress markers and generation of inflammatory cytokines. [8]

Zinc enhances the expression of interleukin-2 and interleukin-2 receptors

Production of interleukin (IL)-2 is decreased in zinc deficient human beings and zinc is essential to IL-2-mediated T-cell activation. We used a human Th(0) malignant lymphoblastoid cell line, HUT-78 to study the effect of zinc on IL-2 production in PHA/PMA activated T-cells. In zinc deficient cells, the gene expression of IL-2 was decreased by 50% compared with that in zinc sufficient cells. The effect of zinc was specific and at the transcriptional level. We also showed a significant effect of zinc on the gene expression of IL-2 receptors alpha and beta. Binding of NF-kappaB (a zinc-dependent transcription factor) to DNA was decreased in zinc deficient cells. Using transfection of expression vectors of anti-sense NF-kappaB p105 (precursor of NF-kappaB p50) in cells, we showed that a decrease in gene expression of IL-2 and IL-2 Ralpha may be partly due to decreased activation of NF-kappaB in zinc deficient cells. Our studies demonstrate for the first time, the role of zinc in gene expression of IL-2 and its receptors in HUT-78 cells. We also document that the binding of NF-kappaB to DNA was adversely affected, thereby decreasing the gene expression of IL-2 and IL-2 Ralpha in zinc-deficient HUT-78 cells. [9]

Correction of interleukin-2 gene expression by in vitro zinc addition

Nutritional deficiency of zinc in humans is widespread in the developing world and a conditioned zinc deficiency is observed in many diseased states the elderly population and pregnant women of both developed and developing nations. It was recently reported that zinc is required for Nuclear Factor-kappaB (NF-kappaB) activation and gene expressions of both interleukin-2 (IL-2) and interleukin-2 receptor alpha (IL-2Ralpha) and beta in HUT-78, a Th0 human malignant lymphoblastoid cell line. In this study, it was reported for the first time that zinc is also required for gene expression of IL-2 and IL-2Ralpha in primary cells. Isolated peripheral blood mononuclear cells (MNCs), from zinc deficient elderly subjects was used for this study. NF-kappaB activation was shown to have decreased in the MNCs from zinc deficient subjects, which was corrected by *in vivo* zinc supplementation. It was further shown that either *in vivo* zinc supplementation or the addition of zinc *in vitro* to MNCs from zinc deficient subjects results in correction of the gene expression of IL-2 and IL-2Ralpha. Therefore, it was proposed that in vitro addition of zinc to MNCs for correction of gene expression of IL-2 in humans may be used as a specific test for zinc deficiency. Although currently no known specific laboratory test exists for the diagnosis of zinc deficiency in humans, the use of correction of IL-2 messenger RNA (mRNA) with in vitro zinc addition to MNCs from zinc-deficient subjects may be very useful. [10]

Zinc attenuates tumor necrosis

The objective of this study was to test the hypothesis that zinc can protect against endothelial dysfunction by interfering with oxidative stress mediated cellular signaling and subsequent inhibition of an endothelial cell inflammatory response. Our approach was to compare alterations on molecular and biochemical levels with changes in endothelial barrier function that occur in zinc deficient conditions.

To investigate the hypothesis, endothelial cells were exposed to zinc deficient media for 2 to 10 days to deplete cellular zinc stores. Following this, half of the groups received zinc supplementation (9.2 microM) for 48 hours. The other half served as zinc deficient controls. These cells were then challenged with tumor necrosis factor alpha (TNF) for varying time periods. Nuclear extracts were prepared from cells and analyzed for nuclear factor kappa B (NF-kappa B) and activator protein-1 (AP-1) binding. Media from cells were analyzed for interleukin 8 (IL-8) production and cellular proteins were determined.

Zinc supplementation resulted in a 74% increase in cellular zinc content. It was also shown that a 1.5 hour exposure to TNF (100 U/mL medium) significantly increased NF-kappa B and AP-1 binding, which was lowered considerably when cells were supplemented with physiological levels of zinc. Zinc supplementation also caused a marked attenuation in IL-8 expression by endothelial cells in response to TNF-mediated cell activation.

The previous data clearly show that zinc is a protective and critical nutrient for maintenance of endothelial integrity. The present data suggest that zinc may protect against cytokine mediated activation of oxidative stress sensitive transcription factors, upregulation of inflammatory cytokines and endothelial cell dysfunction. This may have implications in understanding mechanisms of atherosclerosis. [11]

Effect of Cu supplementation on genomic instability in chemically-induced mammary carcinogenesis

A study assessed the effect of dietary supplementation (copper or copper and resveratrol) on the intensity of carcinogenesis and the frequency of microsatellite instability in a widely used model of mammary carcinogenesis induced in the rat by treatment with 7,12-dimethylbenz[a] anthracene (DMBA).

DNA was extracted from rat mammary cancers and normal tisues, amplified by PCR, using different polymorphic DNA markers and the reaction products were analyzed for microsatellite instability.

It was found that irrespective of the applied diet there was no inhibition of mammary carcinogenesis in the rats due to DMBA. Besides, in the groups supplemented with Cu(II) or Cu(II) and resveratrol, the tumor formation was clearly accelerated. Unlike the animals that were fed with standard diet, the supplemented rats were characterized by the loss of heterozygosity of microsatellite D3Mgh9 in cancer tumors (by respectively 50 and 40%). When the animals received Cu (II) and resveratrol supplemented diet the occurrence of genomic instability was additionally found in their livers in the case of microsatellite D1Mgh6 (which was stable in the animals without dietary supplementation).

Identification of the underlying mechanisms by which dietary factors affect genomic stability might prove useful in the treatment of mammary cancer as well as in the incorporation of dietary factors into mammary cancer prevention strategies. [12]

Effect of Cu(II) coordination compounds on patients with colorectal cancer

Colorectal cancer (CRC) is a serious medical and economical problem of our times. It is the most common gastrointestinal cancer in the world. In Poland, the treatment and detection of CRC are poorly developed and the pathogenesis is still unclear. One hypothesis suggests a role of reactive oxygen species (ROS) in the pathogenesis of CRC. Experimental studies in recent years confirm the participation of ROS in the initiation and promotion of CRC. The aim of the study was to examine the effect of the following coordination compounds coordination compounds: dinitrate (V) tetra-(3,4,5-trimethyl-N1-pyrazole-κN2) copper(II), dichloro di-(3,4,5-trimethyl-N1-pyrazole-κN2) copper(II), dinitrate (V) di-(1,4,5-trimethyl-N1-pyrazole-κN2) copper(II), dichloro di-(1,3,4,5-tetramethyl-N1-pyrazole-κN2) copper(II) on the activity of antioxidant enzymes superoxide dismutase (SOD, ZnCu-SOD) and catalase (CAT) in a group of patients with colorectal cancer (CRC) and in the control group consisting of patients with minor gastrointestinal complaints.

This study was conducted in 20 patients diagnosed with colorectal cancer at the age of 66.5±10.2 years (10 men and 10 women) versus the control group of 20 people (10 men and 10 women) aged 57.89±17.10 years without cancer lesions in the biological material hemolysate prepared in a proportion of 1ml of water per 1 ml of blood. CAT activity was measured by the Beers method [13], while SOD activity was measured by the Misra and Fridovich method. [14]

It was found that patients with CRC showed a statistically significant decrease of SOD and CAT activity (CAT-12,75±1.97 U/g Hb, SOD-1111.52±155.52 U/g Hb) in comparison with the control group (CAT-19.65±2,17 U/g Hb, SOD-2046.26±507.22 U/g Hb). Simultaneously, we observed that the investigated coordination compounds of Cu(II) significantly increased the antioxidant activity of CAT and SOD in patients with CRC (mean: CAT 25.23±4.86 U/g Hb, SOD-3075.96±940.20 U/g Hb).

Patients with colorectal cancer are characterized by reduced activity of antioxidant enzymes catalase and superoxide dismutase which suggests impaired antioxidant barrier. Therefore, coordination compounds of Cu(II), which enhance the activity of CAT and SOD may prove useful in the prevention and treatment of colorectal cancer. [15]

Chemoprevention of carcinogenic progression to esophageal adenocarcinoma by the manganese superoxide dismutase supplementation

Oxidative stress is related to the carcinogenic pathway of reflux esophagitis, to Barrett's metaplasia to esophageal adenocarcinoma (EAC). Recent studies have shown that a decreased manganese superoxide dismutase (MnSOD) level is associated with the increased incidences of Barrett's esophagus (BE) and EAC. The aim of this study was to investigate

MnSOD supplementation as a chemopreventive agent to prevent oxidative injury and subsequent BE and EAC formation.

Our esophagoduodenal anastomotic (EDA) model was done on rats according to our established procedure and treated with Mn(III)-tetrakis(4-benzoic acid) porphyrin (MnTBAP; 10 mg/kg, i.p. every 3 days). Histologic changes were determined after the EDA model at 1, 3, and 6 months. Lipid peroxidation and 8-hydroxy-deoxyguanosine for DNA oxidative damage were determined by the thiobarbituric acid reactive substance assay and immunohistochemical staining. Enzymatic activities of MnSOD and Cu/ZnSOD were evaluated and the rate of proliferation was determined by proliferating cell nuclear antigen staining.

Severe esophagitis was seen in 100% of the EDA rats and morphologic transformation within the esophageal epithelium was observed with intestinal metaplasia (40% of animals) and cancer (40% of animals) identified after 3 months. Decreased oxidative damage, along with the decreased degree of esophagitis and incidence of BE (20%) and EAC (0%) was found in MnTBAP-treated EDA rats comparing with the saline treated EDA control. Decreased proliferation (46%) and increased SOD enzymatic activities (25%) were also found in the EDA rats treated with MnTBAP.

MnTBAP protected rat esophageal epithelium from oxidative injury induced by EDA, and it could prevent the transformation of esophageal epithelial cell to BE to EAC by preservation of antioxidants. [16]

Manganese superoxide dismutase switches cancers between early and advanced stages

Manganese superoxide dismutase (MnSOD) plays a critical role in the survival of aerobic life and its aberrant expression has been implicated in carcinogenesis and tumor resistance to therapy. However, despite extensive studies in MnSOD regulation and its role in cancer when and how the alteration of MnSOD expression occurs during the process of tumor development *in vivo* are unknown. Here we generated transgenic mice expressing a luciferase reporter gene under the control of human MnSOD promoter enhancer elements and investigated the changes of MnSOD transcription using the 7,12-dimethylbenz(α)anthracene (DMBA)/12-O-tetradecanoylphorbol-l3-acetate (TPA) multistage skin carcinogenesis model. The results show that MnSOD expression was suppressed at a very early stage but increased at late stages of skin carcinogenesis. The suppression and subsequent restoration of MnSOD expression were mediated by two transcription-factors, Sp1 and p53. Exposure to DMBA and TPA activated p53 and decreased MnSOD expression via p53-mediated suppression of Sp1 binding to the MnSOD promoter in normal-appearing skin and benign papillomas. In squamous cell carcinomas, Sp1 binding increased because of the loss of functional p53. We used the chromatin immunoprecipitation, electrophoretic mobility shift assay and both knockdown and overexpression of Sp1 and p53 to verify their roles in the expression of MnSOD at each stage of cancer development. The results identify MnSOD as a p53-regulated gene that switches between early and advanced stages of cancer. These findings also provide strong support for the development of means to reactivate p53 for the prevention of tumor progression. [17]

The role of calcium and magnesium

To prospectively evaluate the association of dietary calcium and magnesium intake with cancer incidence and mortality, data of 24,323 participants of the Heidelberg cohort of the European Prospective Investigation into Cancer and Nutrition (EPIC-Heidelberg), who were aged 35-64 years and cancer free at recruitment (1994-1998) were analyzed using multivariate Cox regression models. After an average follow up time of 11 years, 2,050 incident cancers were diagnosed and 513 cancer deaths occurred. Dietary calcium intake was inversely but not statistically significantly associated with colorectal cancer risk (hazard ratio [HR] for per 100 mg increase in intake: 0.95; 95% confidence interval [CI]: 0.88, 1.02) and lung cancer risk (HR for per 100 mg increase in intake: 0.94; 95% CI: 0.87, 1.02). No statistically significant associations were observed between dietary calcium intake and site-specific or overall cancer incidence or mortality. Dietary magnesium intake was not statistically significantly associated with any of the investigated outcomes. This prospective cohort study provides no strong evidence to support that high dietary calcium and magnesium intake in the intake range observed in a German population may reduce cancer incidence or mortality. **[18]**

Biochemical markers in oral carcinogenesis

The development of oral cancer is a multistep process arising from pre-existing potentially malignant lesions. The incidence of Oral Submucous Fibrosis (OSMF) has now taken, particularly targeting the younger generation. Leukoplakia is the most common precancer seen today, probably representing 85% of oral precancer. It has been established by epidemiological studies that over 95% of oral cancers are histologically squamous cell carcinomas. Estimation of trace elements might help in early detection, differential diagnosis and treatment planning of oral premalignant and malignant lesions. Biochemical alterations in the serum of these patients can help to not only in early diagnosis but also as indicators of prognosis for appropriate treatment as the disease progresses. In this study, oral precancer (OSMF/Leukoplakia), cancer and control groups were included.

In this study, serum levels of copper showed gradual increase from precancer to the cancer group as compared to controls which was statistically significant. The present study highlights that high levels of copper in areca nut, a major etiological factor in OSMF plays an initiating role in stimulation of fibrinogenesis by up-regulation of lysyl oxidase. This causes inhibition of degradation of collagen and its accumulation, thereby causing OSMF. The rise in serum copper may be due to increased turnover of ceruloplasmin in the serum of carcinoma patients.

Serum iron levels are considered as biochemical indicators for nutritional assessment. A statistically significant reduction in the serum iron level was present in the precancer group in our study. A decrease in the cancer group but higher than that of precancer group was found to be significant. Utilization of iron in collagen synthesis by the hydroxylation of proline and lysine leads to a decrease in the serum iron levels in OSMF patients. In most cases, clinical anemia may be a contributing factor. Inadequate intake of food due to a burning sensation and vesiculation in the oral cavity might also be an important factor. Reduction in the serum iron level may be due to malnutrition caused by the tumour burden in cancer patients. There appears to be an association between serum iron content and oral carcinogenesis. More detailed studies with more databases should be instituted to elucidate the exact role of iron.

Various epidemiological studies have implicated selenium as a cancer protective agent. Studies indicate that higher dietary intake of selenium in humans may be protective. The serum selenium concentration was found to be decreased in the oral precancer and cancer groups taken in the study. A decrease in the serum selenium level in oral carcinoma patients can be attributed to the protective antioxidant role in cancer. No similar study has been done on serum levels of trace elements (copper, iron and selenium) for oral precancer and cancer. Thus it was conducted for deeper understanding.

An attempt was also made to assess these parameters as predictors for the occurrence and progression of lesions in the decreasing order. It can be suggested that biochemical assessment of oral precancer and cancer patients may help in earlier diagnosis and for prognosis of these lesions. This may also serve in predicting the malignant potential of the premalignant lesions. These efforts may be of value for proactive intervention of high risk groups (potentially malignant conditions and lesions). [19,21-22]

References

[1] Investigation of occupational and environmental causes of respiratory cancers (ICARE): a multicenter, population-based case-control study in France. BMC Public Health. 2011, 11, 928 (10 pages).

[2] Low-dose gallium nitrate for prevention of osteolysis in myeloma: results of a pilot randomized study, Journal of Clinical Oncology 1993, 11(12), 2443-2450.

[3] Oral mucositis prevention by low-level laser therapy in head-and-neck cancer patients undergoing concurrent chemoradiotherapy: a phase III randomized study. International journal of radiation oncology, biology, physics. 2012, 82(1), 270-275.

[4] Zinc in cancer prevention, 2009, 61(6), 879-87.

[5] Influence of extraneous supplementation of zinc on trace elemental profile leading to prevention of dimethylhydrazine-induced colon carcinogenesis. 2010, 20(8), 493-497.

[6] Chemopreventive potential of zinc in experimentally induced colon carcinogenesis. 2007, 171(1-2), 10-18.

[7] In vitro ^{14}C-labeled amino acid uptake changes and surface abnormalities in the colon after 1,2-dimethylhydrazine-induced experimental carcinogenesis: protection by zinc. The Journal of Environmental Pathology, Toxicology and Oncology 2011, 30(2), 103-11.

[8] Zinc in human health: effect of zinc on immuMolecular medicine (Cambridge, Mass). 2008, 14(5-6), 353-357.

[9] Zinc enhances the expression of interleukin-2 and interleukin-2 receptors in HUT-78 cells by way of NF-kappaB activation. Journal of laboratory and clinical medicine. 2002, 140(4), 272-289.

[10] Correction of interleukin-2 gene expression by in vitro zinc addition to mononuclear cells from zinc-deficient human subjects: a specific test for zinc deficiency in humans. Translational Research 2006, 148(6), 325-333

[11] Zinc attenuates tumor necrosis factor-mediated activation of transcription factors in endothelial cells. Journal of the American College of Nutrition. 1997, 16(5), 411-417.

[12] Bobrowska B, Skrajnowska D, Tokarz A. Effect of Cu supplementation on genomic instability in chemically-induced mammary carcinogenesis in the rat. Journal of Biomedical Science 2011, 18, 95 (5 pages).

[13] Beers Jr RF and Sizer IW. A spectrophotometric method for measuring the breakdown of hydrogen peroxide by catalase. Journal of Biological Chemistry 1952, 195, 133-140.

[14] Misra HP, Fridovich I. The role of superoxide anion in the antioxidation of epinephrine and a simple assay for superoxide dismutase. Journal of Biological Chemistry 1972, 247, 3170-3175.

[15] Kubiak K, Malinowska K, Langer E, Kziki C. Effect of Cu(II) coordination compounds on the activity of antioxidant enzymes catalase and superoxide dismutase in patients with colorectal cancer. Polski przeglad chirurgiczny 2011, 83(3), 155-160.

[16] Martin C, Liu B, Wo JM, Ray MB, LI Y. Chemoprevention of carcinogenic progression to esophageal adenocarcinoma by the manganese superoxide dismutase supplementation. Clinical cancer research; an official journal of the American Association for cancer research. 2007, 13(17), 5176-5182.

[17] Dhar SK, Tangpong J, Chaiswing L, Oberley TD, Clair DK. Manganese superoxide dismutase is a p53-regulated gene that switches cancers between early and advanced stages. Cancer research, 2011, 71(21), 6684-6695.

[18] Li K, Kaaks R, Linseisen J, Johrmann S. Dietary calcium and magnesium intake in relation to cancer incidence and mortality in a German prospective cohort (EPIC-Heidelberg). Cancer Causes Control 2011, 22(10), 1375-1382.

[19] Khanna S and Karjodkar FR. Circulating immune complexes and trace elements (Copper, Iron and Selenium) as markers in oral precancer and cancer: a randomised, controlled clinical trial. Journal of Head & Face Medicine, BioMed Central 2006, 2, 33.

[20] Khanna S. Immunological and biochemical markers in oral carcinogenesis: the public health perspective. International Journal of Environmental Research and Public Health 2008, 5(4), 289-293

[21] Khanna S. Artificial intelligence: contemporary applications and future compass. International Dental Journal 2010, 60(4), 269-272.

Role of Trace Elements in the Chemoprevention of Cancer

Dr Sunali Khanna

Dr Vice President, Indian Academy of Oral Medicine & Radiology,
Assistant Professor, Department of Oral Medicine & Radiology
Nair Hospital Dental College, Mumbai-400 008, India

Usually, metals are considered to be naturally occurring elements found in the earth. Similar elements "minerals" too are associated with formation of rocks. In other words, mineral salts constitute rocks. Due to erosion, these are broken into small fragments over millions of years and then mix in the soil. The microbes in the soil utilize these salts and in turn pass them via food chain to the plants that are eaten by animals and humans. [1] Water is also a source of trace elements in plants and animals. [2]

The industrial revolution led to an increase in the use of metals, for example in factories, agriculture and medicine. Earlier effluents and emissions were not as hazardous since population was relatively less. Currently, over population, scarce resources, environmental degradation and human negligence has become a major concern for the medical scientist. This is a serious concern since metals are almost impossible to eliminate because they do not decompose but can "change" in harmful quantity.

Metals normally enter the body through air, food, water or dermal exposure. To exert toxicity, the metal has to cross the plasma membrane and enter the cell. If a metal is in a lipophilic form such as methyl mercury and arsenic compounds, it readily penetrates the membrane. [3] When bound to a protein such as calcium metallothiomein, the metal is actively taken into the cell by endocytosis. [4] Other metals like lead may be absorbed by passive diffusion. [5]

A trace element is defined as an element being present in a biological sample at concentrations below 0.01% wet weight. [6] The body is made up of major elements consisting of hydrogen, nitrogen, carbon, oxygen and minor elements like chlorine, magnesium, calcium, potassium and phosphorous. Trace elements account for less than 1% of all elements. Earlier, they were not easily detected due to analytical techniques being rudimentary as compared to the super specialized techniques of today that can precisely measure their minute amounts or levels. This is how they received the name of "trace elements".

The trace elements can be divided into 3 categories.

- Essential: iron, iodine, zinc, copper, manganese, cobalt, nickel, silicon, molybdenum, fluorine, chromium, selenium, tin and vanadium.
- Possibly essential: arsenic, bromine, strontium, barium.
- Non essential: boron, cadmium, germanium, lead, mercury, aluminium and rubidium.

All trace elements are toxic if ingested at sufficiently high levels and over a long period. A few trace elements like arsenic, lead, cadmium, thallium and mercury exhibit toxicity even at minute concentrations.

Trace elements influence a number of biochemical, physiological and structural processes in human beings. They play a vital role in the activity of a multitude of biological molecules. Trace element deficiencies can result in reduced activity of the enzymes. In some cases, change in enzyme level is of functional significance and may even be the precursor of clinical disease. In other cases, decrease may not be associated with any demonstrable functional effect. [7] However, since each element is related to so many enzymes, deficiency of a single trace element often not associated with any specific clinical manifestation but rather manifests as a combination of various symptoms.

Imbalances of trace elements

Trace element deficiencies and toxicities give rise to profound functional and structural disorders. These disorders range from subclinical and biochemical changes to lethality. Primary deficiencies and toxicities arise mainly from the following sources—diet, excessive exposure to anthropogenic pollutants, altered physiological demands due to ageing, pregnancy, lactation and rapid growth. Living at high altitude can also be a factor. [8] The change in level of the concentration of the trace element in the body leads to biochemical defects, physiological malfunctions and structural disorders.

Copper imbalance

Excessive levels of copper result in adverse effects on liver, kidney, anaemia and immunotoxicity. It causes gastrointestinal distress and irritation to the respiratory tract such as coughing and pulmonary fibrosis.

Zinc imbalance

Zinc deficiency is highly prevalent in the developed countries. Deficiency leads to growth retardation, neuropathy, decreased food intake, diarrhoea, dermatitis, hair loss, bleeding tendency, hypotension, hypothermia, recurrent infection, anorexia, mental lethargy, increased abortion risk and delayed wound healing. Increased levels cause tachycardia, vascular shock, dyspeptic nausea, gastric distress, oliguria, dizziness, taste disorder, dwarfism and reduced reproductive function.

Selenium imbalance

Deficiency causes cardiomyopathy (Keshan disease), chondrodystrophy, myalgia and dandruff and loose skin. Increase in levels lead to selenosis which is associated with alopecia, nail detachment and central nervous system (CNS) disorder.

Iron imbalance

Deficiency causes anaemia, decrease in physical activity, reduction in body temperature, decrease in resistance to infections and increases in absorption of toxic metals. Excessive levels cause vomiting, diarrhoea, diabetes, hemosiderosis, hepatic and renal dysfunction. Overload, that is an excess of total body iron is associated with several chronic diseases such as heart disease. [9]

Chromium imbalance

Chromium deficiency leads to anxiety, attention deficit disorder, hypoglycemia, aortic cholesterol plaque, arteriosclerosis, infertility, decreased sperm count, obesity and depression. Excessive levels cause nausea, peptic ulcer, growth retardation, liver and kidney dysfunction, and cancer.

Nickel imbalance

Deficiency causes reduced growth, low blood glucose levels, abnormal bone growth and poor absorption of ferric ion. Altered calcium metabolism, vitamin B12 and energy nutrients are also affected by nickel deficiency. High levels in diet are associated with an increased risk of thyroid dysfunction, cardiovascular disease and cancer. Long term exposure can cause decreased body weight, heart and hepatic damage, contact dermatitis, bronchial asthma, lung fibrosis, inflammation and renal diseases. [10]

Link of trace elements to cancer

The immune system is the natural mechanism which defends against cancer. The trace elements zinc, selenium, molybdenum and manganese augment this natural mechanism. Normal development and maintenance of the thymus essentially require zinc. It is also essential for the normal bactericidal and phagocyte function of granulocytes. Blood and serum from cancer patients generally show subnormal zinc levels. Deficiency of zinc promotes cancer by inhibiting normal vitamin A, rapid metabolism and DNA repair.

A deficiency in molybdenum has been cited as a possible factor in the causation of oesophageal cancer. It is known to have anti-neoplastic properties and together with manganese prevents the formation of some experimentally induced cancer. Also, the bactericidal actions of antibiotics are augmented by manganese.

Elevated serum copper levels have been described in patients with a variety of carcinomas. Copper is a biological antagonist of vitamin C and zinc. Reviews of the literature emphasize selenium's antioxidant properties, inhibition of tumor growth and inverse epidemiological co-relations with cancer. [11] There is some disagreement over the inhibitory effect of selenium on the growth of tumors. [12] However, this inhibitory effect on growth of tumors has been well documented. [13] On the other hand, some researchers feel that zinc may be a selenium antagonist. [12] Finally, there is evidence against zinc showing that serum zinc is inversely correlated with blood selenium while blood selenium is inversely correlated with cancer. [12]

A deficiency of molybdenum has been cited as a possible factor in the causation of oesophageal cancer. [14] Molybdenum probably exerts its anticancer effect by reducing nitrosamines and their precursors, i.e. nitrates, nitrite and secondary amines in the diet. Molybdenum fertilizer is used in China to reduce nitrates in foods because grain and vegetables are the largest dietary source of the nitrosamine precursor. [15] Molybdenum is the biological antagonist of cancer promoting copper. [16] The same has been reported even in the fetus. [17] An increase in the ascorbic acid content of grains and vegetable is seen to take place with molybdenum fertilizers.

Manganese has been found comparable to molybdenum in its concentration in animal tissues and fluids of all species examined so far. [18] This alters the subcellular distribution of carcinogenic nickel. [19] This particular anti-carcinogenic effect was specifically related to the site of injection rather than systemic causes.

The biological antagonism of copper with anti-carcinogenic molybdenum and zinc suggests excess copper may be cancer hypothesis is supported with research literature. Elevated serum copper levels have been described in lesions like mammary carcinoma, bronchial carcinoma and gastric carcinomas. [20,21] The highest copper levels were associated with metastatic spread of the disease. Copper was significantly concentrated in malignant cervical and endometrial tumors. Copper is concentrated in malignant melanomas. [22]

It is the failure of the immune surveillance system that is central in the development of cancer. Selenium, zinc, molybdenum and manganese are needed for prevention of cancer in a patient and also to increase the chances for natural immunological remission of cancer. Zinc is very necessary in all aspects for generating the immune protection system. Elevated serum copper in contrast in associated with various cancers and probably also increases their incidence in patients.

Chemopreventive protocols

It is recommended that patients should take Vitamin C in dose of 10 to 20 grams per day. Vitamin A is to be given in a dose of 50,000 mcg / day. Vitamin E needs to be given in doses of at least 4000 mcg twice daily. Selenium is at dose of 100 mcg twice a day. Molybdenum is a dose of 500 mcg per day. Manganese in the form of gluconate is to be given as 50 mcg twice a day. Zinc is needed at a dose of 15 mg per day which should be doubled for cancer patients. [23]

References

[1]   Wood JM. Biological cycles for toxic elements in the environment, Science 1974, 183(129), 1049-1052.

[2]   Bryan GW. The effects of heavy metals (other than mercury) on marine and estuarine organisms. Proceedings of the Royal Society, London B: Biological Sciences 1971 177(48),: 389-410.

[3]   Lakowicz J, Anderson C. Permeability to lipid bilayers to methyl—mercury chloride: Qualification by fluorescence quenching of a carbazole-labeled phospholipid. Chemico-Biological Interactions 1980, 30, 309-323.

[4]   Antila E, Mussalo-Rauhamaa H, Kantola M, Atrosi F, Westermarc T. Association of cadmium with human breast cancer. Science of the Total Environment 1996, 186(3), 251-256.

[5]   Karmakar N, Jayaraman G. Linear diffusion of lead in the intestinal wall: a theoretical study. IMA J Math Appl Med Biol 1988, 5(1), 33-43.

[6]   Salonen JT, Tuomainen T-P, Nyyssonen K, Lakka H-M, Punnonen K, British Medical Journal 1998, 317, 727-730.

[7]   Shenkin A (1997) In Ronbeau JL, Rolandelli RH and Saunders WB (Eds.), Micronutrients in Clinical Nutrition. Enteral and Tube feeding (3rd ed.) pp. 96.

[8]   Iyengar GV and Ayengar ARG (1988) Trace elements and human health including effects on high altitude populations, Ambio, 17:31.

[9]   Salonen JT, Nyyssönen K, Korpela H, Tuomilehto J, Seppänen R, Salonen R. High stored iron levels are associated with excess risk of myocardial infarction in eastern Finnish men. Circulation 1992, 86, 803-811.

[10] Antico A and Soana R. Chronic allergic-like dermatopathies in nickel-sensitive patients. Results of dietary restrictions and challenge with nickel salts. Allergy and Asthma Proceedings 1999, 20(4), 235-242.

[11] WHO (1991) Nickel, IPCS (Internal Program for Chemical Safety) Environmental Health Criteria 108, pp-1-383, World Health Organization, Geneva.

[12] Schauzer G: Trace Elements in Carcinogenesis. In Advances in Nutritional Research (Ed) Draper, Plenum Press, London, 1979.

[13] Lafond M: Is the selenium drinking water standard justified? Medical Hypothesis 1979, 5, 877-899.

[14] Greeder G. Factors influencing the inhibitory effect of selenium on mice inoculated with Erhlich ascites tumor cells. Science 1980, 209, 825-827.

[15] Yang CS. Research on esophageal cancer in China. A review. Cancer Research 1980, 40, 2633-2644.

[16] Ward GM. Molybdenum toxicity and hypocuprosis in ruminants. A review. Journal of Animal Science 1978, 4, 1078-1085.

[17] Meinel B, Bode JC, Koenig W, Richter FW. Contents of trace elements in the human liver before birth. Biology of the Neonate 1979, 35, 225-232.

[18] Underwood EJ. Trace elements in human and animal nutrition. Academic Press, Inc. 1977.

[19] Sunderman Jr FW. Effects of manganese on carcinogenicity and metabolism of nickel subsulfide. Cancer Research 1976, 36, 1790-1800.

[20] Kolaric K. Serum copper levels in patients with solid tumours. Tumour 1975, 61, 173-177.

[21] Kelderling W and Sharpf H. Über die klinische Bedeutung der Serumkupfer—und Serumeisenbestimmung bei neoplastischen Krankheitszuständen. Munchener Medizinische Wochenschrift 1954, 95, 437-439.

[22] Bram S. Vitamin C preferential toxicity of malignant melanoma cells. Nature 1980, 284, 629-631.

[23] Braverman BA and Pfeiffer CC. Essential trace elements in cancer. Orthomolecular Psychiatry, 1982, 11(1), 28-41.

The Role of Surfactants in Combating Cancer

[1]Dr Ahmed Alsabagh and [2]Dr Abdelfattah Badawi

[1,2]Professors, Egyptian Petroleum Research Institute, Cairo, Egypt.

Abstract

Improved means of cancer prevention and treatment remain key goals of global health programmes. This is particularly true in Western society, where the elderly represent a large proportion of the population and where the likelihood of tumour development is compounded by risk factors such as poor fibre/high fat diets and environmental pollution. Dietary intervention represents an attractive, non-invasive means of providing anticancer preventative and therapeutic benefits to at-risk individuals. This review focuses on the evidence for anticancer properties of bovine milk and milk-derived components. Evidence of a role for whole milk constituents, as well as purified minor components, in combating tumorigenesis is outlined. Shortcomings in current studies are highlighted and future opportunities for targeted research to characterize important anticancer properties of milk are discussed. [1]

Lipid based formulations

In the recent years, there is a growing interest in the lipid based formulations for delivery of lipophilic drugs. Due to their potential as therapeutic agents, preferably these lipid soluble drugs are incorporated into inert lipid carriers such as oils, surfactant dispersions, emulsions and liposomes. Among these, emulsion forming drug delivery systems appear to be a unique and an industrially feasible approach to overcome the problem of low oral bioavailability associated with Biopharmaceutics Classification System (BCS) class II drugs. Self-emulsifying formulations are ideally isotropic mixtures of oils, surfactants and cosolvents that emulsify to form fine oil-in-water emulsions when introduced in aqueous media. Fine oil droplets would pass rapidly from stomach and promote wide distribution of drug throughout the lower gastrointestinal tract (GIT) and thereby overcome the slow dissolution step typically observed with solid dosage forms. Recent advances in drug carrier technologies have promulgated the development of novel drug carriers such as control release self-emulsifying pellets, microspheres, tablets and capsules that have boosted the use of "self-emulsification" in drug delivery. Different types of formulations and excipients are used in emulsion forming drug delivery systems to enhance the bioavailability of lipophilic drugs. [2]

Prevention of MDR development in leukemia cells by micelle forming polymeric surfactants

Doxorubicin (Dox) incorporated in nanosized polymeric micelles called SP1049C has shown promise as monotherapy in patients with advanced esophageal carcinoma. The formulation contains amphiphilic block copolymers, pluronics that exhibit the unique ability to chemosensitize multidrug resistant (MDR) tumors by inhibiting the P-glycoprotein (Pgp) drug efflux system and enhancing pro-apoptotic signaling in cancer cells. This work evaluates whether a representative block copolymer, Pluronic P85 (P85) can also prevent development of Dox induced MDR in leukemia cells. For *in vitro* studies murine lymphocytic leukemia cells (P388) were exposed to increasing concentrations of Dox with/without

P85. For *in vivo* studies, BDF1 mice bearing P388 ascite were treated with Dox or Dox/P85. The selected P388 cell sublines and ascitic tumor derived cells were characterized for Pgp expression and functional activity (RT-PCR, Western Blot, rhodamine 123 accumulation) as well as Dox resistance (the 3-(4,5-dimethylthiazol-2-yl)-2,5-diphenyltetrazolium bromide assay was used). The global gene expression was determined by oligonucleotide gene microarrays. The results demonstrated that P85 prevented development of MDR1 phenotype in leukemia cells *in vitro* and *in vivo* as determined by Pgp expression and functional assays of the selected cells. Cells selected with Dox in the presence of P85 *in vitro* and *in vivo* exhibited some increases in IC(50) values compared to parental cells but these values were much less than IC(50) in the respective cells selected with the drug alone. In addition to mdr1, P85 abolished alterations of genes implicated in apoptosis, drug metabolism, stress response, molecular transport and tumorigenesis. In conclusion, pluronic formulation can prevent development of MDR in leukemia cells *in vitro* and *in vivo*. [3]

Pluronic block copolymer surfactants mediate overcoming multidrug resistance in tumor cell lines

A significant obstacle for successful chemotherapy with paclitaxel (PTX) is multidrug resistance (MDR) in tumor cells. Micelles and mixed micelles were prepared from pluronic block copolymer P105 or L101 as the PTX delivery systems for overcoming MDR. Both micelle systems were covalently modified with the targeting agent, folic acid to recognize and bind a variety of tumor cells via their surface over expressed folate receptor. There was an increased level of uptake of folate conjugated micellar PTX (FOL-P105/PTX, FOL-PL/PTX) compared to plain micellar PTX (P105/PTX, PL/PTX) in human breast cancer MDR cell sublines, MCF-7/ADR. The uptake of folate conjugated micellar PTX could be inhibited by free folic acid, which suggested that the level of uptake could be mediated by the folate receptor. The cytotoxicity of folate conjugated micellar PTX in the MDR cell culture model was much higher compared with plain micellar PTX or free PTX and the plain micellar PTX also has higher cytotoxicity than free PTX. Overall, the MDR cells are more susceptible to the cytotoxic effects of pluronic micellar PTX than their parental cells. The introduction of folic acid into P105 or PL mixed micelles enhanced the cell killing effect by active internalization. Increased internalization explained the improved cytotoxicity of the FOL-micellar PTX to tumor cells. This suggests that the combined mechanisms of folate mediated active internalization and pluronic mediated overcoming of MDR to be beneficial in treatment of MDR solid tumors by targeting delivery of micellar PTX into the tumor cells where folate receptor is frequently over expressed. This will reduce accumulation of micellar PTX in other tissues or organs and further reduce side effects and toxicities of the drug. [4]

Polymeric surfactants target and overcome multidrug resistance in cancer therapy

Drug carriers tailored to fit the physicochemical properties of anticancer agents and the therapeutic peculiarities of tumor management are envisioned for improving the effectiveness/toxicity ratio of the current treatments. Polymeric micelles are attracting much attention owing to their unique beneficial features:

- core shell structures capable of hosting hydrophobic drugs and raising the apparent solubility in aqueous medium
- sizes adequate for a preferential accumulation (passive targeting) within the tumor and exhibiting enhanced permeability and retention (EPR) effects
- unimers that modulate the activity of efflux pumps involved in MDR.

This report focuses on amphiphilic polyethylene oxide (PEO) and polypropylene oxide (PPO) block copolymers, namely the linear poloxamers (Pluronic® or Lutrol®) and the X-shaped poloxamines (Tetronic®) as components of polymeric micelles able to play the three roles listed above. Specific facets of poloxamers have been highlighted some years ago but recently their wide range of possibilities is beginning to be fully elucidated and understood. Poloxamines are new excipients in the cancer arena and the comparison of their performance with that of poloxamers may enable the identification of aspects of their architecture relevant for the optimization of micellar carriers. Clinical trials in progress indicate that drug loaded polymeric micelles are beneficial with regard to efficiency, safety and compliance of the treatment and quality of life of the patients. The fact that some copolymers are already approved for internal use and several chemotherapy agents will be off patent soon may help to bring the clinical use of poloxamer or poloxamine based micelles into reality in the coming years. [5]

Polymeric surfactants with covalently entrapped cytostatic agents is a system showing strong promise for targeted drug delivery

Doxorubicin (DOX) is clinically applied in cancer therapy but its use is associated with dose limiting severe side effects. Core crosslinked biodegradable polymeric surfactants composed of poly(ethylene glycol)-β-poly([N-(2-hydroxypropyl) methacrylamide lactate] (mPEG-β-p(HPMAm-Lac[n])) diblock copolymers have shown prolonged circulation in the blood stream upon intravenous administration and enhanced accumulation in tumors through the enhanced permeation and retention (EPR) effect. However a physically entrapped anticancer drug (paclitaxel) was previously shown to be rapidly eliminated from the circulation, likely because the drug was insufficiently retained in the micelles. To fully exploit the EPR effect for drug targeting, a DOX methacrylamide derivative (DOX-MA) was covalently incorporated into the micellar core by free radical polymerization. The structure of the doxorubicin derivative is susceptible to pH-sensitive hydrolysis enabling controlled release of the drug in acidic conditions (in either the intratumoral environment and/ or the endosomal vesicles). Some 30-40% w/w of the added drug was covalently entrapped and the micelles with covalently entrapped DOX had an average diameter of 80 nm. The entire drug payload was released within 24 h incubation at pH 5 and 37 °C, whereas only around 5% release was observed at pH 7.4. DOX micelles showed higher cytotoxicity in B16F10 and OVCAR-3 cells compared to DOX-MA, likely due to cellular uptake of the micelles via endocytosis and intracellular drug release in the acidic organelles. The micelles showed better antitumor activity than free DOX in mice bearing B16F10 melanoma carcinoma. The results presented in this paper show that mPEG-b-p(HPMAm-Lac(n)) polymeric micelles with covalently entrapped doxorubicin is a system with high promise for the targeted delivery of cytostatic agents. [6]

Block copolymer surfactants for cancer therapy

The main objective of this study was to develop and characterize a pH-responsive and biodegradable polymeric surfactants as a tumor targeting drug delivery system. The pH responsive block copolymer was synthesized by a Michael type step copolymerization of hydrophilic methyl ether poly(ethylene glycol) (MPEG) with a pH-responsive and biodegradable poly(beta-amino ester) resulting in an amphiphilic MPEG-poly(beta-amino ester) block copolymer. This copolymer, which formed nano sized self-assembled micelles under aqueous conditions, could be efficiently (74.5%) loaded with doxorubicin (DOX) using a solvent evaporation method. In an *in vitro* drug release study, these DOX-loaded polymeric micelles showed noticeable pH dependent micellization-demicellization behavior, with rapid release of DOX from the micelles in weakly acidic environments (pH 6.4) but very slow release under physiological conditions (pH 7.4). Moreover, due to demicellization, the tumor cell uptake of DOX released from polymeric micelles was much higher at pH 6.4 than at pH 7.4. When *in vivo* antitumor activity of pH responsive polymeric micelles was evaluated by injecting the DOX-loaded polymeric micelles into B16F10 tumor bearing mice, these micelles notably suppressed tumor growth and also prolonged survival of the tumor bearing mice, compared with mice treated with free DOX. [7]

Block copolymer surfactants enhanced drug delivery to human glioma cells

A new type of block copolymer micelles for pH triggered delivery of poorly water soluble anticancer drugs has been synthesized and characterized. The micelles were formed by the self assembly of an amphiphilic diblock copolymer consisting of a hydrophilic polyethylene glycol (PEG) block and a hydrophobic polymethacrylate block (PEYM) bearing acid labile ortho ester side chains. The diblock copolymer was synthesized by atom transfer radical polymerization (ATRP) from a PEG macro-initiator to obtain well defined polymer chain length. The PEG-β-PEYM micelles assumed a stable core shell structure in aqueous buffer at physiological pH with a low critical micelle concentration as determined by proton NMR and pyrene fluorescence spectroscopy. The hydrolysis of the ortho ester side chain at physiological pH was minimal yet much accelerated at mildly acidic pH. Doxorubicin (Dox) was successfully loaded into the micelles at pH 7.4 and was released at a much higher rate in response to slight acidification to pH 5. Interestingly, the release of Dox at pH 5 followed apparently a biphasic profile consisting of an initial fast phase of several hours followed by a sustained release period of several days. Dox loaded in the micelles was rapidly taken up by human glioma (T98G) cells *in vitro* accumulating in the endolysosome and subsequently in the nucleus in a few hours, in contrast to the very low uptake of free drug at the same dose. The dose dependent cytotoxicity of the Dox loaded micelles was determined by the MTT assay and compared with that of the free Dox. While the empty micelles themselves were not toxic, the IC(50) values of the Dox loaded micelles were approximately ten times (by 24h) and three times (by 48h) lower than the free drug. The much enhanced potency in killing the multidrug resistant human glioma cells by Dox loaded in the micelles could be attributed to high intracellular drug concentration and the subsequent pH triggered drug release. These results establish the PEG-β-PEYM block copolymer with its acid labile ortho ester side chains as a novel and effective pH responsive nanocarrier for enhancing the delivery of drugs to cancer cells. [8]

Polyethylene glycol-block-poly-4-vinylbenzylphosphonate and cationic surfactants as highly stable, pH responsive drug delivery systems

A new family of block ionomer complexes (BIC) formed by polyethylene glycol-block-poly-4-vinylbenzylphosphonate (PEG-β-PVBP) and various cationic surfactants was prepared and characterized. These complexes spontaneously self assembled in aqueous solutions into particles with average size of 40-60nm and remained soluble over the entire range of the compositions of the mixtures including stoichiometric electro neutral complexes. Solution behavior and physicochemical properties of such BIC were very sensitive to the structure of cationic surfactants. Furthermore, such complexation was used for the incorporation of cationic anticancer drug, doxorubicin (DOX) into the core of BIC with high loading capacity and efficiency. The DOX/PEG-β-PVBP BIC also displayed high stability against dilution and changes in ionic strength. Furthermore, DOX release at the extracellular pH of DOX/PEG-β-PVBP BIC was slow. It was greatly increased at the acidic pH mimicking the endosomal/lysosomal environment. Confocal fluorescence microscopy using live MCF-7 breast cancer cells suggested that DOX/PEG-b-PVBP BICs are transported to lysosomes. Subsequently, the drugs are released and exert cytotoxic effect killing these cancer cells. These findings indicate that the obtained complexes show promise as attractive candidates for delivery of cationic drugs to tumors [9].

Micellar nanoparticles as a new therapeutic approach for patients with ovarian cancer

Micellar nanoparticles based on linear polyethylene glycol (PEG) block dendritic cholic acids (CA) copolymers (telodendrimers) for the targeted delivery of chemotherapeutic drugs in the treatment of cancers are reported. The micellar nanoparticles have been decorated with a high affinity "OA02" peptide against α-3 integrin receptor to improve the tumor targeting specificity which is overexpressed on the surface of ovarian cancer cells. Click chemistry was used to conjugate alkyne containing the OA02 peptide to the azide group at the distal terminus of the PEG chain in a representative PEG(5k)-CA(8) telodendrimer (micelle forming unit). The conjugation of OA02 peptide had negligible influence on the physicochemical properties of PEG(5k)-CA(8) nanoparticles. It was hypothesized that the OA02 peptide dramatically enhanced the uptake efficiency of PEG(5k)-CA(8) nanoparticles (NP) in SKOV-3 and ES-2 ovarian cancer cells via receptor mediated endocytosis but not in α-3 integrin negative K562 leukemia cells. When loaded with paclitaxel,

OA02-NPs showed significantly higher *in vitro* cytotoxicity against both SKOV-3 and ES-2 ovarian cancer cells as compared with non targeted nanoparticles. Furthermore, the *in vivo* biodistribution study showed OA02 peptide greatly facilitated tumor localization and the intracellular uptake of PEG(5k)-CA(8) nanoparticles into ovarian cancer cells as validated in SKOV3-luc tumor bearing mice. Finally, paclitaxel (PTX) loaded OA02-NPs exhibited a superior antitumor efficacy and a lower systemic toxicity profile in nude mice bearing SKOV-3 tumor xenografts when compared with equivalent doses of non-targeted PTX-NPs as well as clinical paclitaxel formulation (Taxol). Therefore, OA02-targeted telodendrimers loaded with paclitaxel have great potential as a new therapeutic approach for patients with ovarian cancer. **[10]**

Intelligent polymeric micelles for cancer therapy

Recent efforts are carried out for the design and preparation of intelligent polymeric micelles from functional polyethylene glycol-polyamino acid (PEG-PAA) block copolymers. The polymeric micelles feature a spherical sub-100 nm core shell structure in which anticancer drugs are loaded avoiding undesirable interactions *in vivo*. Chemical modification of the core forming block of PEG-PAA with a hydrazone linkage allows the polymeric micelles to release drugs selectively at acidic pH (4-6). Installation of folic acids on the micelle surface improves cancer cell specific drug delivery efficiency along with pH controlled drug release. These intelligent micelles appear to have superiority over classical micelles that physically incorporate drugs. Studies showed both controlled drug release and targeted delivery features of the micelles reduced toxicity and improved efficacy significantly. Further developments potentiate combination delivery of multiple drugs using mixed micelles. Therefore clinically relevant performance of the polymeric micelles provides a promising approach for more efficient and patient-friendly cancer therapy [11].

Surfactant prevention of compliations from cancer

Polyethylene glycol (PEG) is a clinically widely used agent with profound chemopreventive properties in experimental colon carcinogenesis. Over the past several years, Corpert et al. have indicated that polyethylene glycol (PEG) has remarkable efficacy as a chemopreventive agent. [12,13] Indeed, the ability of this novel agent to suppress tumors or aberrant crypt foci in the azoxymethane (AOM) treated rat model was > 90%, generally out performing reported efficacies of nonsteroidal anti-inflammatory drugs or that of other known chemopreventive agents. [14] Previous studies have suggested that PEG is a remarkably potent chemopreventive agent with effects seen throughout the spectrum of carcinogenesis. Specifically, PEG has been shown to cause regression of established lesions such as aberrant crypt foci [15] and also inhibit the earliest stages of colon carcinogenesis including at the predysplastic mucosa. [16] Recently, it was found that epidermal growth factor receptor (EGFR) is the proximate membrane signaling molecule through which PEG initiates antiproliferative activity with snail/β-catenin pathway playing the central intermediary function. [17] Tween 80 is described as a nonionic, surface active detergent, polyoxyethylene sorbitan monooleate. Tween 80 and some other nonionic and ionic surfactants appear to increase permeability of the cell membrane and to enhance uptake of dyes and proteins. [18-19] Tween 80 enhance uptake of the antibiotics AD and DM, especially in drug-resistant cells, as demonstrated by radioautography and as suggested by growth response in combination experiments [20] Tween-80 has been shown to potentiate the cytotoxicity of etoposide (VP16) against several human lung adenocarcinoma cells by increasing the accumulation of Vp16 in vitro. Tween-80 mediated sensitization of lung adenocarcinoma cell to Vp16 is considered to be related to both the characteristics of the cell membrane in adenocarcinoma cells and the lipotropic properties of Vp16. These results suggest this combination might have the potential to improve the therapeutic index of Vp16 in human lung adenocarcinoma. [21] The nonionic detergent Tween 80, which is used as a solvent for lipophilic drugs such as VP-16 and Taxotere, was found to reverse VP-16 resistance of the P-glycoprotein associated multidrug resistance phenotype via increasing VP-16 influx. In adriamycin resistant human chronic myelogenous leukemia K562 cells (K562/ADM), which overexpress mdr1 mRNA, the accumulation of VP-16 was only about 10% that in wild-type K562 cells. Tween 80 enhanced VP-16 accumulation in K562/ADM cells but did not influence VP-16 accumulation in parental K562 cells. VP-16 efflux was rapid and similar in both sensitive and resistant cell lines and was not blocked by Tween 80 or verapamil. Under glucose free conditions, VP-16 accumulation in K562/ADM cells was only half of that in K562 cells. Tween 80 increased VP-16 accumulation in K562/ADM cells in glucose-free medium. In growth inhibition assay, Tween 80 reversed K562/ADM sensitivity to VP-16 without cell damage. Taken together, Tween 80 reverses VP-16 sensitivity in multidrug resistant K562 cells by increasing inclux, which is considered to be the primary mechanism of VP-16 resistance in K562/ADM-cells. [22].

References

[1]   Harsharnjit S. Gill and M. L. Cross. Anticancer properties of bovine milk. British Journal of Nutrition (2000), 84, Suppl. 1, S161-S166

[2]   Wadhwa J, Nair A, Kumria R. Emulsion forming drug delivery system for lipophilic drugs. Acta Poloniae Pharmaceutica 2012, 69(2), 179-191.

[3]   Sharma AK, Zhang L, Li S, Kelly DL, Alakhov VY, Batrakova EV. Prevention of MDR development in leukemia cells by micelle-forming polymeric surfactant. Journal of congrolled release; official journal of the Controlled Release Society. 2008, 131(3), 220-227.

[4]   Wang Y, Yu L, Han L, Sha X, Fang X. Difunctional pluronic copolymer micelles for paclitaxel delivery: synergistic effect of folate-mediated targeting and pluronic-mediated overcoming multidrug resistance in tumor cell lines. International journal of pharmaceutics. 2007, 337(1-2), 63-73.

[5]   Lorenza B, Sosnik A, Concheiro A. PEO-PPO block copolymers for passive micellar targeting and overcoming multidrug resistance in cancer therapy. Current Drug Targets 2011, 12(8), 1112-30.

[6]   Talelli M, Iman M, Varkouhi AK, Rijcken CJ, Schiffelers RM, Etrych T, Ulbrich K. Nostrum C. Lammers T, Storm G, Hennink WE. Core-crosslinked polymeric micelles with controlled release of covalently entrapped doxorubicin. Biomaterials, 2010, (30), 7797-7804.

[7]   Ko J, Park K, Kim YS, Kim MS, Han JK, Kim K, Park RW, Kim IS, Song HK, Lee DS, Kwon IC. Tumoral acidic extracellular pH targeting of pH-responsive MPEG-poly(beta-amino ester) block copolymer micelles for cancer therapy. Journal of controlled

relsease; official journal of the Controlled Release Society, 2007, 123(2), 109-115.

[8] Tang R, Ji, W, Panus D, Palumo RN, Wang C. Block copolymer micelles with acid-labile ortho ester side-chains: Synthesis, characterization, and enhanced drug delivery to human glioma cells. Journal of controlled relesase; official journal of the Controlled Release Society 2011, 151(1), 18-27.

[9] Kamimura M, Kim JO, Kabanov AV, Bronich TK, Nagasaki Y. Block ionomer complexes of PEG-block-poly(4-vinylbenzylphosphonate) and cationic surfactants as highly stable, pH responsive drug delivery system. Journal of controlled release: official journal of the Controlled Release Society 2012, 160(3), 486-494.

[10] Xiao K, Li Y, Lee JS, Gonik AM, Dong, T, Fung G, Sanchez E, Xing L, Cheng HR, Luo J, Lam BA. OA02 peptide facilitates the precise targeting of paclitaxel-loaded micellar nanoparticles to ovarian cancer in vivo. Cancer research. 2012, 72(8), 2100-2110.

[11] Bae Y, Kataoka K. Intelligent polymeric micelles from functional poly(ethylene glycol)-poly(amino acid) block copolymers. Advanced drug delivery reviews. 2009, 61(10), 768-784.

[12] Roy HK and Koetsier JL. Chemoprevention of colon carcinogenesis by polyethylene glycol: suppression of epithelial proliferation via modulation of snail/β-catenin signaling. Molecular Cancer Therapeutics 2006, 5, 2060-2069.

[13] Wali RK, Dhananjay P, Kunte JK, Koetsier MB, Hemant KR. Polyethylene glycol-mediated colorectal cancer chemoprevention: roles of epidermal growth factor receptor and snail. Molecular Cancer Therapy 2008, 7(9), 3103-3111.

[14] Höber R and Höber J. The influence of detergents on some physiological phenomena, especially on the properties of the stellate cells of the frog liver. Journal of General Physiology 1942, 25, 705-715.

[15] Hoders M, Palmer CG, Warren A. The effect of surface active agents on the permeability to dye of the plasma membrane of Ehrlich Ascites cells. Experimental Cell Research 1960, 21, 164-169.

[16]   Kay ERM. The effects of Tween 80 on the in vitro metabolism of cells of the Ehrlich—Lettré ascites carcinoma. Cancer Research 1965, 25, 764-769.

[17]   Malenkov A, Bogatyreva SA, Bozhkova VP, Modjanova EA, Vasiliev JM. Reversible alterations of the surface of ascites tumor cells induced by a surface-active substance, Tween 60. Experimental Cell Research 1960 1967, 48, 307-318.

[18]   Miller GW AND Janicki BW. Further studies on selective cytotoxicity of Triton WR-1339. Cancer Chemotherapy Reports 1968, 52, 243-249.

[19]   Palmer CG, Hodes ME, Warren AK. The action of synthetic surfactants on membranes of tumor cells. I. Morphological observations. Experimental Cell Research 1961, 24, 429-439.

[20]   Riehm H and Biedler JL. Potentiation of drug effect by Tween 80 in Chinese hamster cells resistant to actinomycin D and daunomycine. Cancer Research 1972, 32, 1195-1200.

[21]   Tsujino I, Yamazaki T, Masutani M, Sawada U, Horie T. Effect of Tween-80 on cell killing by etoposide in human lung adenocarcinoma cells. Cancer Chemotherapy and Pharmacology 1999, 43(1), 29-34.

[22]   Yamazaki T, Sato Y, Hanai M, Mochimaru, Tsujio I, Sawada U, Horie Y. Non-ionic detergent Tween 80 modulates VP-16 resistance in classical multidrug resistant K562 cells via enhancement of VP-16 influx. Cancer Letters 2002, 28, 149(1-2), 153-161.

Amino Acids, Peptides, Proteins and Metals in the War against Cancer

Dr David RK Harding

Professor of Chemistry, Institute of Fundamental Sciences, Massey University Palmerston North, New Zealand

Abstract

The studies in this report on the effectiveness of amino acids and their polymeric forms for combating and reversing cancer cell growth. Amino acids, peptides and protein, with and without carrying metal ions offer much potential in the war against cancer. Amino acids enjoy the capability of therapeutic effect via all administration routes, including oral and the first pass effect via the liver. The polymeric forms of amino acids are restricted to non-gastric routes.

Introduction

This chapter looks at a selection of amino acids and their polymeric forms—polyamino acids, peptides and proteins—and their involvement in preventing and/or fighting cancer. The role of amino acids, peptides and proteins that are involved in nutraceutical and metal carrying therapies for cancer treatment will be discussed.

Amino acids, peptides and proteins play a significant part in the war against cancer in mammals. Their actions vary from direct involvement in cellular metabolism to drug delivery of non-amino acid containing anti-cancer agents. Their roles vary from metal transporters to cell necrosis agents themselves to drug delivery. One approach to cancer therapy advocates the reduction of amino acid intake in the diet. Suitable peptides can be radiolabelled to act anti-cancer agents that can be tracked throughout the body. Various amino acids are reported as having beneficial effects in cancer treatment. Foods rich in some amino acids are recommended by many. Some large proteins have anticancer activity.

Mammalian amino acids in the prevention/ control of carcinogenesis

The best cure for curing cancer is prevention. However we cannot avoid breathing, eating and touching at risk. The action of amino acids and their derivatives can be harmful or helpful. For example, the amino acids phenylalanine (Phe) and tyrosine (Tyr) as well as L-glutamine (Gln) and L-methionine (Met) are reported to support tumour growth. [1] In this study two prostate cancer cell lines (DU145 and PC3) and two normal cell lines (human infant foreskin fibroblast and human prostate epithelial cells) were used to study the effects of these four amino acids. All four amino acids inhibited DU145 and PC3 cell growth. Lack of Met, Tyr and Phe induced apoptosis in DU145, whereas only deprivation of Met caused cell death in PC3 cells. The healthy cells showed restricted growth in this study but did not exhibit cell death due to the reduction of these amino acids. Implications were that healthy humans can exist for at least four weeks on a diet deficient of these amino acids. The results point to the potential for dietary amino acid restriction in cancer prevention and therapy. In another study Epner et al. showed a positive effect of reducing Met intake in terminal patients suffering from prostate cancer. [2] Arginine restriction has also been indicated as a positive indicator for cancer control particularly for melanoma, hepatocellular carcinoma, some mesiotheliomas and some renal cell cancers—cell lines that cannot produce arginine. [3]

On the other hand, the amino acid derivative N-acetyl-L-cysteine (NAC), an anti-oxidant, shows much promise for antitumor therapy. Extending a previous study that showed cigarette smoke produced lung cancer in new born mice, Balansky et al. showed that mice treated with NAC during pregnancy produced much healthier young that than those in the control group. [4] This study appears to be the first study to indicate the potential for antioxidant intake during pregnancy that may well reduce the induction of carcinomas from birth at least in the lung.

Thus indications are that dietary amino acid control has its place in cancer prevention and therapy.

L-methionine and L-cysteine also have received much attention as metal coordinating agents and hence become delivery agents to the carcinogenesis sites as a result. For example, L-methylcysteine is combined with selenium to give L-methylselenocysteine (MSC) for use as an anti-cancer agent. [5] Selenium is an essential dietary component that shows strong positive indications as to cancer prevention or control. It is carried through the body bound to Met and Cys in proteins. It can be found in the active sites of proteins including enzymes and can thus prevent cancer development and prevention. However at high levels selenium can become toxic and produce DNA damage. High levels of selenium can inhibit repair proteins by binding to the Cys residues in the protein. Nevertheless selenocysteine and selenomethionine are dietary constituents and available as dietary supplements. Again dietary control is important.

In another study with dietary MSC, NMU-induced mammary cancer in rats was significantly reduced in rats fed MSC compared with the control animals. [6] Of significant importance, this study also produced the first mechanistic link between chemoprevention and circadian rhythm.

Other bioorganic metallic anticancer agents involving amino acids include platinum, palladium, ruthenium, germanium and gold.

In the case of platinum, a study comparing dicarboxylic acids—oxalic, malonic, succinic—with amino acids alanine, valine, tyrosine as platinum-platinum bridging linkers. The linker is an important component of these bridged platinum (II) bridged complexes. Cytotoxicity studies revealed that overall the dicarboxylic acids were better. [7] However this study employed D,L amino acids. No mention was made of using solely L-amino acids.

Another study compared Pt(II) and Pd(II) amino acid complexes as [M(dipyridyl)amino acid where M is Pt or Pd and the amino acids glycine or L-alanine in the anionic form. [8] Against the P388 lymphocytic leukemia cell line, the efficacy studies revealed ID_{50} values as follows: the Pt/Pd-alanine < cis-platin < Pt/Pd-glycine.

Ruthenium (II) cymene complexed with gylcine, D or L-alanine D or L-phenylalanine and L-proline showed lack of activity against A2780 ovarian cancer cells. [9] The paper nevertheless offers further possibilities for the study of Ru-amino acid complexes.

Germanium has been complexed with L-histidine, L-methionine, L-lysine, and L-arginine. [10] In vitro testing against Ehrlich ascites carcinoma (EAC) revealed that the germanium-L-histidine complex showed high cytotoxicity, L-methionine and L-lysine showed moderate activity with arginine a poor last.

Gold nanoparticles (AuNP, 2nm) have been functionalized with a dodecapeptide, PMI (p12, $L-NH_2$-TSFAEYWNLLSP-NH_2) a therapeutic peptide and L-CRGDK a targeting peptide. [11] The targeting peptide increased intracellular uptake of the AuNP most likely due to the high binding of the peptide to the targeted cell receptor (Nrp-1) which is over expressed in cancer cells. Improved delivery of the P12 therapeutic peptide in the cells was also achieved.

Unnatural amino acids in the prevention/control of carcinogenesis

Two examples of unnatural (non-mammalian) amino acids reveal the breadth of the world of "amino acids". 5-Aminosalicylic acid (5-ASA) one might say is an analog of glycine whereas (+)-monascumic acid and (-)-monascumic acid, with their 4 membered ring system have little resemblance to mammalian amino acids.

In one study 5-ASA was conjugated to ursodeoxycholic acid (UDCA, 3α, 7β-dihydroxy-5β-cholan-24-oic acid) and fed to rats with induced colon carcinoma. [12] The efficacy of this diet was compared to that of rats fed with UDCA or 5-ASA alone. The tumour populations were as follows: UDCA-5-ASA 48%, UDCA 56%, 5-ASA 64%, control 84%. In other words, both UDCA and 5-ASA produced lower populations of tumours as well as smaller tumours. Evidence was presented to show that the conjugate was cleaved in the colon. In addition, the adenocarsomas were restricted to the mucosa and sub-mucosa. A continuation of this programme revealed that 5-ASA when injected directly into the lumen of the rats' colon gave a considerable reduction in the incidence of colon cancer that was chemically induced by N-methylurea.

In another rat colon tumour study, the prodrug balsalazide (BSZ, (E)-5-([4-(2-carboxyethylcarbamoyl) phenyl]diazenyl)-2-hydroxybenzoic acid)—as its disodium salt—was tested as a chemo-preventative of tumours in B6-Min/+ mice. BSZ showed a dose dependent protective effect by reducing cellular proliferation and inducing apotosis. [13]

Monascumic acid (syn-2-isobutyl-4-methylazetidine-2,4-dicarboxylic acid) variants can be isolated from fermented rice. [14] They are actually imino acids (like proline, Pro). The rice used was the red mold rice *Manascus pilosus*. (+)-Monoascumic acid and (-)-monascumic acid showed moderate inhibition on NOR 1 induced carcinomas pointing to chemoprevention possibilities—again possible therapy with a foodstuff.

Polyamino acids

Yet another aspect of the range of options offered by amino acids in cancer therapy is found in the capabilities of single amino acids when polymerised. Examples of polyamino acids that are in various stages of clinical trial are as follows:

- polyglutamic acid as a polymer conjugate will carry paclitaxel (Taxol, $(2\alpha,4\alpha,5\beta,7\beta,10\beta,13\alpha)$-4,10-bis(acetyloxy)-13-{[(2R,3S)-3-(benzoylamino)-2-hydroxy-3-phenylpropanoyl]oxy}-1,7-dihydroxy-9-oxo-5,20-epoxytax-11-en-2-yl benzoate) for treatment of lung, breast, head, neck cancer, advanced Kaposki's sarcoma and campothecin (broad spectrum)
- polyglutamic acid-polyethylene glycol as micelles will carry cis-platin (broad spectrum anti-cancer) and oxaliplatin (colorectal cancer)
- polylysine in a polyamino-dendritic form will transport MUC-1 peptide (anti-cancer vaccine). [15]

Polyamino acids are nontoxic and biocompatible. They offer a range of polymer sizes with at least twenty options when considering natural mammalian amino acids only. Not only do polyamino acids offer the multidrug carrying capabilities they also can be focussed on improving drug uptake and/or stimulating responsiveness. To date, polyamino acids have been used in various forms varying from polymer conjugates to micelles, nanoparticles, dendrimers, physical mixtures (vaccines), vesicles, capsules and fibres. The versatility they offer (charged, polar, non-polar) has made them a serious component of anti-cancer research and hopefully soon therapy.

Peptides and proteins in the chemoprevention of chemically induced carcinogenesis

Peptides and proteins, largely polymers of natural amino acid, in many cases, in addition to their natural action/s, can be modified to other applications.

Radioactive metal complexes of DOTA (1,4,7,10-tetraazacyclododecane-1,4,7,10-tetraacetic acid) with peptides have become popular for targeted imagining and anti-tumour therapy as well as being used as MRI contrast agents. [16] One example of this is somatostatin (SS-14, SST) growth hormone release inhibiting hormone, a dodecapeptide with the following sequence H-Ala-Gly-Cys$_3$-Lys-Asn-Phe-Phe-Trp-Lys-Thr-Phe-Thr-Ser-Cys$_{14}$-OH. The cysteines at the 3 and 14 positions allow for a cyclic form of this peptide. It has a short *in vivo* half-life of 1.82 minutes such that even though it has a many interesting actions it is of little use in therapy. Somatostatin controls (suppresses) the release of growth hormone, thyrotropin (TRH, thyroid releasing hormone), insulin and gut hormones. Many analogs have been synthesised since 1973, some with the insertion in some case of D-amino acids to extend the half-life. Analogs of SST such as octreolide, lanreolide and vapreotide have been use in cancer therapy to suppress the over production of the above hormones in tumours. [17-19]

One family of analogs is based on the octreotide peptide, H-D-Phe-Cys-Phe$_3$-D-Trp-Lys-Thr-Cys-Thr(ol), where again a cyclic form is possible and the CV-terminal threonine carboxyl terminus is reduced to the alcohol. As for many somatostatin analogs, D-tryptophan was used to extend half-lives. Ginj et al. have developed a number of radiolabelled octapeptide analogs of the octreotide family. [17] In their study, a segment of somatostatin with a phenylalanine (Phe$_3$) has been substituted with unnatural amino acids. Of 24 analogs studied, they found 2 DOTA-[1-NaI$_3$]-octatreptide and DOTA-[BzThi]-octreotide had significantly broader affinity for the cell surfaces of the cell lines they studied when the DOTA peptides carried ^{111}In, ^{90}Y, and [68]GA. Their studies show a distinct place for somatostatin in the world of cytotoxic agents for targeted delivery of radioactive materials to cells with small peptides. In another more recent study, a somatostatin tyrosine-3-octreotide was incorporated in radiolabelled (indium-111) nano particles (liposomes/micelles). [20] This initial study showed promise for the labelled liposomal nano particles. Although the authors state much more needs to be done their study points the way to visualising malignant tumours.

Human **bradykinin** (BK), a nonapeptide with the sequence is reported to be a vasodilator that dilates all blood vessels including those in tumours and hence also contributes to tumour growth. [21] The BK nonapeptide amino acid sequence can be altered to produce peptide analogs that reverse BK's activity and show promise for human lung and prostate cancers. [22] In one study, BK analogs were shown to be less toxic and more effective in suppressing human small cell lung cancer cell growth in mice than the well known anti-cancer agent, cis-platin. [23]

One of the themes that run throughout anti-cancer therapy is dietary intake—in short the food we eat and the foods we can eat. Carcinogenesis arises from both environmental and hereditary factors. Those who have a high intake of soyabean foods in their diet have lower rates of carcinogenesis and death resulting from cancer. An example of is an anticancer agent in soya bean appears to a peptide of 43 amino acids. The peptide, lunasin (43 amino acid peptide) shows much promise for anti-tumour therapy. [24,25] Although found first in soyabean, it was also later found in wheat, barley and other grains. To date it has shown strong promise in vitro against colon, breast and prostate cancers. *In vivo* studies are currently being carried out. In its 43 amino acid sequence, this peptide to date exhibits a segment that delivers lunasin into the cells, a segment that targets histones (very basic proteins) in the cells and a highly acidic segment that binds to chromatin (a DNA/protein chromasomal complex in cell nuclei).

Another recent example of peptide-anticancer activity is found in soricidin, a 54 amino acid peptide. [26] Soricidin was isolated from the submaxilary saliva gland of the Northern Short-tailed Shrew (Blarina brevicauda). It is claimed to be useful in preventing/treating cancers resulting from over expression of calcium channels in the intestine. However the parent, soricidin, also has paralysing activity. Stewart and co-workers discovered that the paralysing site in the soricidin sequence was remote from the calcium inhibiting site. [26] Indeed the peptide and analogs they produced had increased calcium channel blocking capabilities greater than soricidin itself in some cells. The peptides also had increased solubility, increased shelf life and reduced antigenicity.

Bovine lactoferrin has been studied for its potential as an anti-carcinogenic and anti-metastastic agent with colon studies proving the most promising to date. Lactoferrin like many proteins is a multifunctional protein (glycoprotein) of 80kDa. [27,28] Although it can now be produced recombinantly it is readily isolated from normal milk as bovine lactoferrin (bLF). Human colostrum has the highest concentration of lactoferrin followed by bovine milk. Lactoferrin is also found in tears, saliva, seminal and uterine secretions. It has antifungal and antibacterial activity that is especially helpful in newborns. Its overall function is as an immunoprotector. It carries iron in the blood and not only controls iron blood levels it is active in delivering iron to cells. It can also bind zinc, copper and other metals. In addition to its antibacterial and antifungal activities, lactoferrin shows antiviral, , catalytic, anti-cancer, anti-allergic and radioprotecting functions.

Tsuda et al have investigated the anticancer effects of bLF and have found that it and a 25 amino acid fragment (BLFcin) that has no iron binding capability have anticancer capability against chemically induced cancer in the mouse. [29] In particular promising indications are directed at colon cancer as well as to a lesser extent other cancers in the entire GIT tract and the lungs and liver. Indications are that the protein and its peptide inhibit enzymes and stimulate natural killer cells in the small intestine and blood.

A lactoferrin fragment L12 (amino acids 14-31) has also been fused with elastin-like polypeptide (ELP) to improve its delivery to tumour sites while reducing its adverse side effects on normal tissue and poor plasma kinetics. [30] The fusion was achieved recombinantly with L12 fused to the C-terminus of the ELP and a transduction fragment of the HIV-1 Tat protein fused to the N-terminus of the ELP (Tat-ELP-L12). The *in vitro* studies showed that the Tat-ELP-L12 complex showed promising anti-solid tumour potential for this delivery system.

TRAIL (tumour necrosis factor-related apoptosis-inducing ligand) induces tumour cell death but does not harm normal cells. [31] It is a protein of 281 amino acids in length and behaves as a transmembrane protein. Trimers of TRAIL bind to cancer cell receptors to a. induce apoptosis and b. block anti-apoptosis action. Kedinger et al. have set up a model mouse model. The mouse TRAIL protein has some 65% homology with the human proteins. Transgenic mice were bred to over express TRAIL in the basal level of the epidermis and the claim TRAIL is *not toxic and does not interfere with the normal development and/or homeostasis of skin.* TRAIL mice showed delayed tumour development, reduced tumour numbers and a high percentage of benign tumours as compared to the control animals.

Summary

This short report has highlighted some approaches to the use and potential of amino acids and their derivatives in the world wide effort to the beat cancer. The spectrum of this approach is considerable and ranges from a molecular weight ranges for very low to over one hundred thousand, a full hydrophilicity-lipophilicity range of polarities and functional goups. As discussed above, foodstuffs provide many possibilities for delivering these preventative and/or therapeutic natural cancer preventative agents to the body.

References

[1] Fu Y-M, Yu Z-X, Li Y-Q, Ge X, Sanchez PJ, Fu X, Meadows GG, Meadows G. Specific amino acid dependency regulates invasiveness and viability of androgen-independent prostate cancer cells. Nutrition and Cancer 2003, 45(1), 60-73.

[2] Lu S, Chen GL, Chengyi R, Kwabi-Ado B, Epner DE. Methionine restriction selectivity targets thymidylate synthase in prostate cancer cells. Biochemical Pharmacology 2003, 66, 791-800.

[3] Fuen L, You M, Wu CJ, Kuo MT, Wangpaichitr S, Savaraj N. Arginine deprivation as a target therapy for cancer. Current Pharmaceutical Design 2008, 14, 1049-1057.

[4] Balansky R, Ganchev G, Iltcheva M, Steele VE, De Flora S. Prenatal N-acetylcysteine prevents cigarette smoke-induced lung cancer in neonatal mice. Carcinogenesis 2009, 30(8), 1398-1401.

[5] Letavayová L, Vlčková V, Brozmanová J. Selenium: From cancer prevention to DNA damage. Toxicology 2006, 227, 1-14.

[6] Zhang X and Zarbl H. Chemopreventive doses of methylselenocysteine alter circadian rhythm in rat mammary tissue. Cancer Prevention Research 2008, 1(2), 119-127.

[7] Zhang J, Li Y, Sun J, Li W, Gong Y, Zheng X, Cui J, Wang R, Wu J. Synthesis, cytotoxicity and DNA-binding levels of new type binuclear platinum(II) complexes. European Journal of Medicinal Chemistry 2009, 44, 4772-4777.

[8] Paul AK, Mansuri-Torshizi H, Srivastava TS, Chavan SJ, Chitnis MP. Some potential antitumor 2,2'-dipyridylamine Pt(II)/Pd(II) complexes with amino acids: their synthesis, spectroscopy, DNA binding, and cytotoxic studies. Journal of Inorganic Biochemistry 1993, 50, 9-20.

[9]   Habtermariam A, Melchart M, Fernández R, Parsons R, Oswald IDH, Parkin A, Fabbiani FP, Davidson JE, Dawson A, Aird RE, Jodrell DI, Sadler PJ. Structure-activity relationships for cytotoxic ruthenium (II) arene complexes containing N,N-, N,O-, and O,O-chelating ligands. Journal of Medicinal Chemistry 2006, 49, 6858-6868.

[10]   Ismail DA and Noaman E. Synthesis and antitumour activity of four germanium amino acid complexes. Egyptian Journal of Chemistry 2007, 50(1), 29-37.

[11]   Kumar A, Ma H, Zhang X, Huang K, Jin S, Liu J, Wei T, Cao W, Zou G, Liang X-J. Gold nanoparticles functionalized with therapeutic and targeted peptides for cancer treatment. Biomaterials 2012, 33, 1180-1189.

[12]   Narisawa T and Fukaura Y, Prevention by intrarectal 5-aminosalicylic acid of N-methylnitrosourea-induced colon cancer in F344 rats. Disease of the Colon & Rectum 2003, 46(7), 900-903.

[13]   MacGregor DJ, Kim YS, Sleisenger MH, Johnson LK. Chemoprevention of colon cancer carcinogenesis by balsalazide: inhibition of azoxymethane-induced aberrant crypt formation in the rat colon and intestinal tumor formation in the B6-Min/+ mouse. International Journal of Oncology 2000, 17(1), 173-179.

[14]   Akihisha T, Mafune S, Ukiya, Kimura Y, Yasukawa K, Suzuki T, Tokuda H, Tanabe N, Fukuoka T. (+) and (-)-syn-2-Isobutyl-4-methylazetidine-2,4-dicarboxylic acids from the extract of *Monascus pilosus*-fermented rice (Red-Mold rice). Journal of Naturak Products 2004, 67, 479-480.

[15]   González-Aramundiz JV, Lozano MV, Sousa-Herves A, Fernandez-Megia E, Csaba N. Polypeptides and polyaminoacids in drug delivery. Expert Opinionon Drug Delivery 2012, 9(2), 183-201.

[16]   De León-Rodríguez LM, Kovacs Z. The synthesis and chelation chemistry of DOTA-peptide conjugates. Bioconjugate Chemistry 2008, 19(2), 391-402.

[17]   Ginj M, Schmitt JS, Chen J, Waser B, Reubi J-C. de Jong M, Schulz S, Maecke HR. Design, synthesis, and biological evaluation

of somatostatin-based radiopeptides. Chemistry & Biology 2006, 13, 1081-1090.

[18] Grimberg A. Somatostatin and cancer: applying endocrinology to oncology. Cancer Biology & Therapy 2004, 8, 731-733.

[19] Froideveaux S and Eberle AN. Somatostatin analogs and radiopeptides in cancer therapy. Biopolymers 2002, 66(30), 161-183.

[20] Helbok A, Rangger C, von Guggenberg E, Saba-Lepek M, Radolf Ing T, Thurner G, Andreae F, Prassl R. Decristoforo C. Targeting properties of peptide-modified radiolabeled liposomal nanoparticles Nanonmedicine: Nanotechnology, Biology and Medicine 2012, 8(1), 112-118.

[21] Iyer AK, Khaled G, Fang J, Maeda H. Exploiting the enhanced permeability and retention effect for tumour targeting. Drug Discovery Today 2006, 11(17/18), 812-818.

[22] Stewart JM, Gera L, Chan Jr DC, Bunn PA, York EJ, Simkeviciene V. Helfrich B. Bradykinin-related compounds as new drugs for cancer and inflammation. Canadian Journal of Physiology and Pharmacology 2002, 80, 275-280.

[23] Gera L, Chan DC, Helfrich B, Bunn Jr B, Paul A, York EJ, Eunice J, Stewart JM. Bradykinin-related compounds having anti-cancer activity in vivo superior to cisplatin and SU5416. Peptides 2000, Proceedings of the European Peptide Symposium, 26th, Montpellier, France, Sept. 10-15, 2000, (2001), Meeting Date 2000, 637-638. Publisher: Editions EDK, Paris, Fr.

[24] Hernández-Ledesma B, de Lumen BO, Lunasin. A novel cancer preventive seed peptide. Perspectives in Medicinal Chemistry 2008, 2, 75-80.

[25] Hernández-Ledesma B, Hsieh C-C, de Lumen BO. Lunasin. A novel seed peptide for cancer prevention. Peptides 2009, 30, 426-430.

[26] Stewart JM. Soridicin peptide composition for cancer treatment by inhibiting TRPV6 calcium channel activity. PCT Int. Appl., WO 20091149343, (2009) 82 pages.

[27] Wiki en.wikipedia.org/wiki/Lactoferrin

[28]   Adleroval L, Bartoskoval A, Faldyna M. Lactoferrin: a review. Veterinarni Medicina 2008, 53(9), 457-468.

[29]   Tsuda H, Fukamachi K, Xu J, Sekine K, Ohkubo S, Takasuka N, Iigo M. Prevention of carcinogenesis and cancer metastasis by bovine lactoferrin. Proceedings of the Japanese Academy of Sciences 2006, B82, 208-215.

[30]   Massodi I, Thomas E, Raucher D. Application of thermally responsive elastin-like polypeptide fused to a lactoferrin-derived peptide for treatment of pancreatic cancer. Molecules 2009, 14, 1999-2015.

[31]   Kedinger V, Muller S, Gronemeyer H. Targeted expression of tumor necrosis factor-related apoptosis-inducing ligand TRAIL in skin protects mice against chemical carcinogenesis. Molecular Cancer 2011, 10(34) online—http://www.molecular-cancer.com/content/10/1/34.

www.ingramcontent.com/pod-product-compliance
Lightning Source LLC
Chambersburg PA
CBHW020911290526
45784CB00002BA/504